SECOND EDITION

SPORT STRETCH

MICHAEL J. ALTER, MS

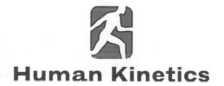

Human Kinetics

Library of Congress Cataloging-in-Publication Data

Alter, Michael J., 1952-
    Sport stretch / Michael J. Alter. -- 2nd ed.
      p.   cm.
    Includes bibliographical references.
    ISBN 0-88011-823-7
    1. Physical education and training.   2. Stretching exercises.
  I. Title.
  GV711.5.A45   1997
  613.7'1--dc21   97-14591
                                               CIP

ISBN: 0-88011-823-7

Acquisitions Editor: Martin Barnard; **Developmental Editor:** Julie Rhoda; **Assistant Editor:** Sandra Merz Bott; **Editorial Assistants:** Jennifer Jeanne Hemphill and Laura T. Seversen; **Copyeditor:** Barbara Field; **Proofreader:** Karen L. Bojda; **Graphic Designer:** Robert Reuther; **Graphic Artist:** Denise Lowry; **Photo Editor:** Boyd La Foon; **Cover Designer:** Jack Davis; **Photographer (cover):** Anthony Neste; **Illustrators:** Michael Richardson and Keith Blomberg; **Printer:** United Graphics

Illustrations on pp. 79, 84, 101, 114, 128, 137, 155, 178, 181, 189, 194, and 210 © K. Galasyn-Wright, Champaign, IL, 1994.

Human Kinetics books are available at special discounts for bulk purchase. Special editions or book excerpts can also be created to specification. For details, contact the Special Sales Manager at Human Kinetics.

Printed in the United States of America   10 9 8 7 6

Human Kinetics
Web site: www.humankinetics.com

United States: Human Kinetics, P.O. Box 5076, Champaign, IL 61825-5076
800-747-4457
e-mail: humank@hkusa.com

Canada: Human Kinetics, 475 Devonshire Road, Unit 100, Windsor, ON N8Y 2L5
800-465-7301 (in Canada only)
e-mail: hkcan@mnsi.net

Europe: Human Kinetics, P.O. Box IW14, Leeds LS16 6TR, United Kingdom
+44 (0) 113 278 1708
e-mail: humank@hkeurope.com

Australia: Human Kinetics, 57A Price Avenue, Lower Mitcham, South Australia 5062
08 8277 1555
e-mail: liahka@senet.com.au

New Zealand: Human Kinetics, P.O. Box 105-231, Auckland Central
09-523-3462
e-mail: hkp@ihug.co.nz

To my developmental editors, Sue Wilmoth Savage, Holly Gilly, and Julie Rhoda, without whose assistance this book and those preceding it would not have been possible.

CONTENTS

Preface vi
Acknowledgments vii

Part I UNDERSTANDING FLEXIBILITY 1

The Benefits of Stretching 2
How the Body Responds to Stretching 2
What Happens When You Stretch? .10
Stretching Techniques 11
What Causes Muscle Soreness? 17
Appropriate Injury Management 20
Adding a Stretching Program to Your Workout 21
The Controversy About Stretching .24
Advanced Stretches 25

Part II ALL-STAR STRETCHES **29**

12 All-Star Stretches 30
28 Maximal Isolation All-Stars 32

Part III STRETCHING ROUTINES FOR SPECIFIC SPORTS **37**

Archery 38
Baseball, Softball, and Cricket (General Field Players) 39
Baseball, Softball (Pitchers), and Cricket (Bowlers) 40
Basketball 41
Bowling 42
Cross-Country Skiing 43
Cycling and Triathlon 44
Dance (Beginning) 45
Dance (Advanced) 46
Diving (3- to 10-Meter) 47
Figure Skating 48
Football (Offensive Line and Defensive Line) 49

Football (Defensive Backs and Receivers) 50
Golf 51
Gymnastics 52
Hiking and Backpacking 53
Ice Hockey 54
In-Line Skating 55
Jogging 56
Lacrosse 57
Martial Arts (Beginning) 58
Martial Arts (Advanced) 59
Race Walking 60
Rowing, Kayaking, and Canoeing 61
Sailing and Windsurfing 62
Skiing (Alpine) 63
Soccer (International Football) 64
Squash 65
Swimming 66
Table Tennis 67
Tennis, Racquetball, and Handball 68
Track and Field (High Jump and Pole Vault) 69
Track and Field (Hurdles, Long- and Triple-Jumps, and Sprints) .70
Track and Field (Discus, Hammer Throw, Javelin, and Shot Put) .71
Volleyball 72
Water Skiing 73
Weight Lifting 74
Weight Lifting (Very Light Weights) .75
Wrestling 76

Part IV ILLUSTRATED INSTRUCTIONS FOR 311 STRETCHES 77

Feet and Ankles 79
Lower Legs 84
Hamstrings 101
Adductors 114
Quadriceps 128
Hips and Gluteals 137
Lower Torso 155
Upper Back 178
Neck 181
Pectorals 189
Shoulders 194
Arms and Wrists 210

References 219
About the Author 223

PREFACE

Flexibility is one of several important components of physical fitness and successful performance in disciplines ranging from archery to volleyball to martial arts to football. Your body is your instrument; athletes and the coaches, trainers, therapists, and physicians who work with them should take advantage of every opportunity, therefore, to develop optimal flexibility. The purpose of this second edition of *Sport Stretch,* like the first edition, is to help athletes and their coaches reduce the risk of athletic injury and improve sport performance by incorporating a flexibility training program within their established training program.

This second edition has been substantially improved over the first edition. Changes include

- updated and expanded information on muscle structure and muscle soreness as they relate to flexibility and stretching,
- an illustrated list of 12 *all-star* stretches for the whole body that you can incorporate into your flexibility training program every day,
- 12 additional sport-specific stretching routines (41 total sport-specific routines),
- a list of the best single stretches for 28 muscle groups, and
- 27 new illustrated stretches (311 total).

Whether you're a dancer, pitcher, swimmer, or high jumper, you can improve your flexibility safely and effectively using the programs in this book. With over 300 stretching exercises, this book provides the most comprehensive selection of stretches of any book devoted to the topic of sport-specific stretching. I wish you much success with your individual sport endeavors and hope the information and stretches provided in this edition of *Sport Stretch* help you achieve your sport-specific potential.

ACKNOWLEDGMENTS

I wish to express my gratitude to the many who made this work possible. First, I wish to acknowledge Martin Barnard, acquisitions editor at Human Kinetics, for encouraging the project and contributing ideas to enhance the final product.

Second, I wish to acknowledge the patience, skill, loyal support, and assistance of developmental editor Julie Rhoda who had the task of directing and managing the project. Julie was also the developmental editor of *Science of Flexibility* (1996), and it was again a pleasure to hear her soft-spoken, warm, and encouraging voice.

I am once again indebted to the excellent work of artist Michael Richardson who drew all of the stretching exercises that appeared in the first edition. Keith Blomberg added the new illlustrations and modified several previous drawings for this second edition, and these contributions are also appreciated.

In addition, I extend my gratitude to the companies, publishers, and authors who granted permission to reproduce drawings, photographs, and other illustrative material. In particular, my thanks go to Appleton & Lange; Human Kinetics; Little, Brown and Company; Gerald H. Pollack, PhD; Universal Gym Equipment, Inc.; and VCH Publishers.

Last, I wish to acknowledge the efforts of production director Ernie Noa, production manager Judy Rademaker, graphic designer Bob Reuther, graphic artist Denise Lowry, assistant editor Sandra Merz Bott, editorial assistants Jennifer Hemphill and Laura Seversen, and all the other members of the Human Kinetics staff for their helpfulness throughout the production of this book.

PART I

UNDERSTANDING FLEXIBILITY

Flexibility is the ability to move muscles and joints through their full ranges of motion. Throughout this text, the term *flexibility* refers to the degree of "normal" motion. In contrast, stretching refers to the process of elongating connective tissues, muscles, and other tissues. Flexibility and stretching exercises fall into several basic categories depending on the manner in which a muscle is stretched. Several of these more common flexibility categories are as follows:

1. Static flexibility relates to range of motion (ROM) about a joint with no emphasis on speed during stretching; hence, static flexibility is the result of static stretching. A common example is a "split."

2. Ballistic flexibility is usually associated with bobbing, bouncing, rebounding, and rhythmic motion. In ballistic stretching, momentum of a moving body or limb is used to increase the ROM forcibly. Consequently, the risk of injury is greater. An example of a ballistic stretch is swinging your arms out to the side so that the momentum is responsible for the increased ROM.

3. Dynamic or functional flexibility refers to the ability to use a range of joint movement in the performance of a physical activity at either normal or rapid speed. In contrast to ballistic stretching, it includes no bouncing or jerky movements. Dynamic or functional flexibility directly corresponds to the specificity of the stretching process as it relates to the activity. Dynamic or functional flexibility has the highest correlation to sport achievement.

4. Active flexibility refers to a range of motion accomplished by the voluntary use of one's muscles without assistance. An example of active flexibility is an athlete slowly raising and holding the kicking leg to a 100-degree angle. Active flexibility may be static or dynamic.

Research has proven that flexibility does not exist as a general characteristic but is specific to a particular joint and joint action (Merni et al. 1981); that is, range of motion is specific to each joint in the body. For instance, an athlete may be flexible in the hips but tight in the shoulders, or tight in the right hip but flexible in the left hip. Attempts to correlate flexibility to body proportions, body surface area, skinfold, and weight have yielded inconsistent results (Alter 1996).

A review of the literature (Alter 1996) demonstrates that flexibility is specific to a given group of sports as well as to a given joint, a given side, and a given speed. Even within sport groups, particular patterns of flexibility are related to frequent or unique joint movements in those activities, events, or positions. For example, a baseball pitcher's dominant shoulder possesses an increased range of external rotation over his other shoulder (Cook et al. 1987). Earlier research found that throwing velocity was significantly related to the range of external shoulder rotation (Sandstead 1968). Similarly, Cohen et al. (1994) demonstrated that numerous flexibility measures— including dominant wrist flexion, dominant shoulder forward flexion, and dominant shoulder internal rotation at zero degrees of abduction—are directly related to tennis serve velocity. Therefore, flexibility training focusing on improving a joint's ROM must be specifically tailored to the needs of the individual athlete and the sport in which he or she is participating.

BENEFITS OF STRETCHING

- Stretching can optimize an athlete's learning, practice, and performance of many types of skilled movements. For example, a high jumper using the straddle technique requires additional flexibility in the adductors, groin, and hamstrings.
- Stretching can increase an athlete's mental and physical relaxation.
- Stretching can promote development of body awareness.
- Stretching can reduce risk of joint sprain or muscle strain.
- Stretching can reduce risk of back problems.
- Stretching can reduce muscle soreness.
- Stretching can reduce the severity of painful menstruation (dysmenorrhea) for female athletes.
- Stretching can reduce muscle tension.

THE BENEFITS OF STRETCHING

Flexibility is developed when connective tissues and muscles are elongated through regular, proper stretching. In contrast, flexibility diminishes over time when these tissues are not stretched or exercised. Some of the many reasons why athletes should want to improve their flexibility through stretching exercises are listed to the left.

However, stretching is only beneficial when done properly. For example, athletes need to make stretching a regular part of their training program and devote several minutes to stretching each day to see results. Athletes also need to stretch gradually, slowly, and using the correct technique to avoid injuring themselves during stretching. Just as there is more than one way to achieve a set goal, there is more than one stretch to enhance flexibility. The 311 stretching exercises detailed in part IV of this book allow you to add variety to your stretching routine.

HOW THE BODY RESPONDS TO STRETCHING

Two of the many intricate parts that make up the human body are the skeletal and the muscular systems. Your bones help make up the specialized support system of your body's skeleton, and to perform their support function, they must be held together. Joints are points at which two or more bones connect, and the connections are performed primarily by ligaments and assisted by muscles and tendons.

Muscle Structure

The primary function of muscle tissue is to produce movement through its ability to contract and develop tension. Muscles are attached to bone by tendons. The place where a muscle attaches to a relatively stationary point on a bone is called the origin, and the end of the muscle that moves with the bone is known as the insertion. When a muscle contracts, it develops tension that is transmitted to the bones by the tendons, and movement takes place; thus, movement is caused by the interaction of the muscular and skeletal systems.

Muscles are obviously important to stretching and developing flexibility. Muscles come in various shapes and sizes, but all are composed of progressively

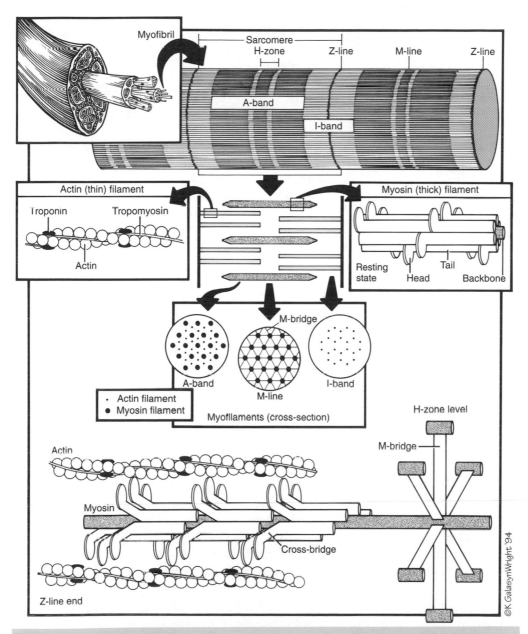

Figure 1 Organization of skeletal muscle tissue from the gross to the molecular level.
© K. Galasyn-Wright, Champaign, IL, 1994.

smaller units (figure 1). The *myofibrils* are the elements of your muscles that contract (shorten), relax, and elongate (stretch) and are composed of functional units or muscle cells called *sarcomeres* which are represented in figure 1 as repeating light and dark patterns. Sarcomeres were originally thought to be composed primarily of just thick (myosin) and thin (actin) filaments, but the existence of a third connecting filament (titin) is now recognized. Electron microphotographs clearly demonstrate the presence of these and other structures (figure 2).

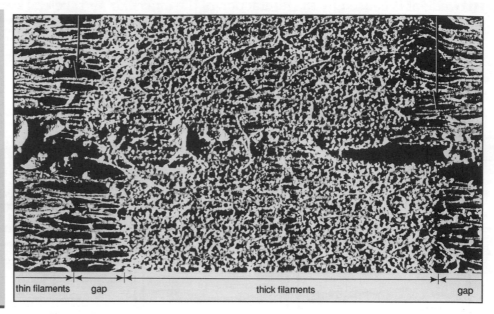

Figure 2 Examples of connecting filaments (titin) in overstretched frog muscle, prepared by freeze-fracture, deep-etch method. Thick filaments (center) do not terminate; they give way to thinner connecting filaments (arrows), which run out of the field toward the Z-line. Thin filament tips, seen at edges of figure, do not overlap the thick filaments.

Reprinted, with permission, from G.H. Pollack, 1990, *Muscles and molecules: Uncovering the principles of biological motion*. (Seattle: Ebner & Sons), 70.

A diagrammatic summary of the sarcomere's principal structures is shown in figure 3. These filaments and structures are significant because they determine how sarcomeres elongate and consequently influence an athlete's flexibility. It is important to understand that the most important component of muscle related to flexibility is the connective tissue that envelops and surrounds the muscle at its various levels of organization.

At present, muscles are hypothesized to function in a way partly described by Huxley's sliding filament theory (Huxley and Hanson 1954). Basically, the muscle fibers receive a nerve impulse that causes the release of calcium ions stored in the muscle. In the presence of adenosine triphosphate (ATP), the "fuel" of the muscles, the calcium ions bind with the actin and myosin filaments to form an electrostatic bond. The bond can be likened to two opposing magnets attracting each other. As a result of this bond, the muscle fibers shorten and develop tension. When the muscle fibers no longer receive nerve impulses, they relax. The recoil of the elastic elements restores the filaments to their former uncontracted lengths.

In contrast, when the muscles are stretched, the actin and myosin reverse the interlinking effect that takes place during contraction. Research has demonstrated that, at first, stretch comes easily to the actin and myosin filaments. As stretch continues, the titin filament takes up more and more of the displacement; hence, the titin filament is primarily responsible for the sarcomere's extensibility and resistance to stretch. This resistance is called "resting tension." If stretching continues, eventually the sarcomere's integrity is compromised and it ruptures.

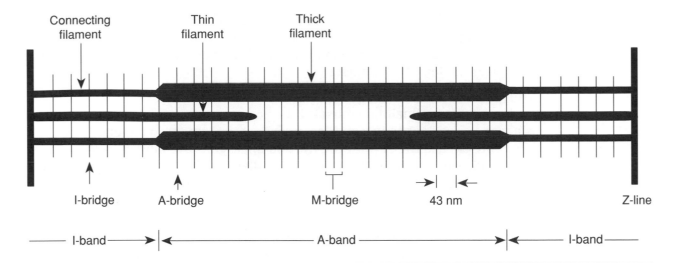

Figure 3 Diagrammatic summary of the sarcomere's principal structures.
Reprinted, with permission, from G.H. Pollack, 1990, *Muscles & molecules: Uncovering the principles of biological motion.* (Seattle: Ebner & Sons), 81.

Research has demonstrated that a sarcomere can be stretched to 150 percent of its resting-state length (Wang et al. 1991). Obviously, then, the contractile elements (filaments) of the sarcomere cannot be a limiting factor in flexibility when the muscle is relaxed. This degree of potential sarcomere elongation is significant for all athletes whose sports require an enhanced range of motion. Thus, if the muscle is relaxed (and there is no structural limitation), and if the connective tissues are properly stretched, virtually any athlete can achieve even a full split. Although this degree of flexibility is not required of most sports, many disciplines require one to possess such a capacity (e.g., gymnastics, figure skating, the martial arts). Keep in mind that the most important component related to flexibility is the connective tissue that envelops and surrounds the muscle at its various levels of organization (i.e., muscle fiber, bundle, and whole muscle). This tissue consists of the endomysium, perimysium, and epimysium, explored later in this section.

Skeletal (voluntary) muscles possess two distinct types of nerve-fiber receptors: the Golgi tendon organs (GTOs) and muscle spindles. These receptors are important because they can sense stretch. The GTOs are located almost exclusively at muscle-tendon or muscle-aponeurosis junctions and not within tendons. An aponeurosis refers to the tendinous sheaths that usually extend along and deep into the belly of the muscle. The GTOs monitor all degrees of muscle tension but are most sensitive to tension forces generated by muscle contraction. Consequently, this monitoring is extremely relevant for specific stretching techniques that use contractions of the muscle being stretched (i.e., proprioceptive neuromuscular facilitation [PNF], described later). Extremely intense stretching is necessary to activate GTOs.

Muscle spindles are miniature muscle fibers and nerve endings in a fusiform-shaped spindle encapsulated by a sheath of connective tissue that run parallel to the muscle fiber. These smaller muscle fibers are referred to as *intrafusal* because of their location within the spindle. The muscle spindles have two types of sensory endings: primary and secondary. Primary endings respond to both a phasic (dynamic) and tonic stretch response. In contrast, secondary endings respond only to tonic stretch. A phasic response measures the length plus rate or velocity of the stretch; hence, such responses play a vital role during ballistic or dynamic stretching. In contrast, the tonic response measures the length of a muscle.

The Stretch Reflex.   The stretch reflex is a basic operation of the nervous system that helps maintain muscle tone and prevent injury. The stretch reflex is a muscle's response to a sudden, unexpected increase in its length. Stretching a muscle lengthens both the muscle fibers and the muscle spindles, and this change in shape of the muscle spindles results in firing of the stretch reflex. The muscle that is being stretched contracts to minimize the increase in its length.

A classic example of the stretch reflex is the knee jerk, or patella reflex. When the patella (kneecap) tendon is given a light tap, the muscle spindles that run parallel to the muscle fibers are stretched and change shape, causing the muscle spindles to fire. This sends a message to the spinal cord. Completing the reflex arc, the spinal cord sends an impulse to the quadriceps (thigh muscles) and causes them to contract; the quadriceps shorten, taking the tension off the muscle spindles.

Beginning athletes generally should avoid strenuous ballistic or bouncing types of stretches, because this type of stretching increases the likelihood of injury and soreness and makes muscular tension increase in the very muscle you are attempting to stretch. This tension makes it more difficult to stretch connective tissues. Hence, for the safest stretching, relax the parts of the muscle that perform contraction and employ slow or static stretching to reduce the probability of initiating the stretch reflex. However, for most sports, ballistic or dynamic stretching is an essential component of the training regime. This topic is discussed below.

Reciprocal Innervation.   Muscles usually operate in pairs of agonists and antagonists, so that when one set of muscles is contracting, the opposing muscles are relaxing. The muscles most directly involved in bringing about a movement are called the agonists or prime movers. Muscles that slow down or oppose the prime movers are called antagonists. The grouping of coordinated and opposing agonistic and antagonistic muscles is called reciprocal innervation. For example, when you flex your arm at the elbow by contracting your biceps, your triceps muscle, which normally extends your arm at the elbow, must relax. If it didn't, the two muscles would be pulling against each other, preventing movement. Similarly, the biceps muscle must relax when you attempt to extend your arm.

Reciprocal innervation is accomplished by cooperation between the nerves supplying any antagonistic pair of muscles. When one of the pair receives an impulse to contract, the other relaxes because it does not receive an impulse to cause contraction. It is therefore inhibited at the same time that its opposing muscle contracts. By taking advantage of this phenomenon, you can induce relaxation in the muscles you want to stretch. For example, to stretch your hamstrings, contract your quadriceps while in a modified hurdler's stretch (see part IV, stretch # 50). Reciprocal innervation will make your hamstrings relax. Consequently, you should feel greater ease as you lean forward into the stretch.

The Inverse Myotatic Reflex.   Perhaps you have experienced a sudden and involuntary relaxation of your muscles when stretching. This is due to the inverse myotatic reflex. The GTOs were thought to be solely responsible for this reflex; however, today we believe that the GTOs along with other receptors are involved in this reflex (Moore 1984).

The GTOs are thought to operate in the following manner. When the intensity of a muscular contraction or stretch on a tendon exceeds a certain critical point, an immediate reflex occurs to inhibit the muscular contraction. As a result, the muscle immediately relaxes and the excess tension is removed. This reaction is possible only because the impulses of the GTOs are powerful enough to override the excitatory impulses of the muscle spindles. This relaxation is a protective mechanism—a safety device to prevent tendons and muscles from being injured by tearing away from their attachments.

However, this system is not fail-safe. We know that the effects of the GTOs can be counterbalanced by additional signals from higher centers of the central nervous system. This process of minimizing the influence of GTOs is referred to as disinhibition of the agonist motoneurons and is a result of athletic training (Brooks and Fahey 1987). The purpose of disinhibition is to push performance to the limits of tissue capacity. In extreme cases, disinhibition in activities such as wrist wrestling and weight lifting can result in torn muscles or tendons.

The inverse myotatic reflex has two important implications for stretching. First, it may explain why, when an athlete is attempting to maintain a stretching position that develops considerable tension in the muscle, a point is suddenly reached where the tension dissipates and the muscle can be stretched even farther. Second, by using a stretching strategy called the contract-relax technique (explained below), relaxation can be induced in muscles that are being stretched. For example, stretch a limb or muscle to the point where further motion in the desired direction is prevented by the tension of the antagonistic muscle. At this point, gradually build to a less than maximal contraction in the stretched muscles (antagonists) for 6 to 15 seconds. This will cause the GTOs to fire and initiate the inverse myotatic reflex. Then, move the joint through the gained range of joint motion. (Note, however, that there is greater risk with this procedure because it develops more tension in the muscle, which may result in soreness and injury.)

Connective Tissue

Connective tissue, which binds together to support the various structures of the body, is the body's most abundant tissue. Its functions include defense, protection, storage, transportation, and general support and repair.

Two types of connective tissue can significantly affect an athlete's range of motion: collagenous connective tissue and elastic connective tissue. The former is composed primarily of collagen and the latter of elastic tissue. Where collagenous fibers dominate, range of motion is restricted. Conversely, a dominance of elastic fibers allows a greater range of motion. Within limits, through flexibility training or rehabilitation, an athlete's tissues can be modified and their performance enhanced.

Technically, the term fascia designates all fibrous connective tissues not otherwise specifically named. Muscle fascia (sheaths) envelop and bind muscle fibers into separate groups. These sheaths are the endomysium, perimysium, and epimysium (figure 4). A muscle's resistance to stretch originates in the meshwork of these connective tissues; as you stretch, your connective tissues become more taut.

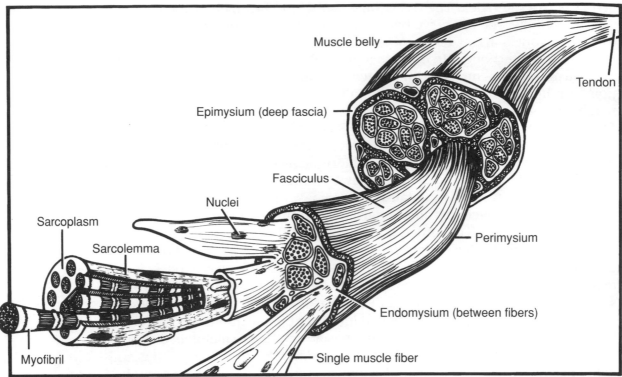

Muscle belly

Tendon

Epimysium (deep fascia)

Fasciculus

Nuclei

Perimysium

Sarcoplasm

Sarcolemma

Endomysium (between fibers)

Myofibril

Single muscle fiber

©K GalasynWright '94

Figure 4 Schematic drawing of a muscle illustrating three types of connective tissue: epimysium (the outer layer), perimysium (surrounding each fasciculus, or group of fibers), and endomysium (surrounding individual fibers).

© K. Galasyn-Wright, Champaign, IL, 1994.

Of great interest to all athletes is the relative importance of various tissues in joint stiffness. The joint capsule (the sacklike structure that encloses the ends of bones) and ligaments are the most important factors, accounting for 47 percent of stiffness, followed by the muscle's fascia (41 percent), the tendons (10 percent), and the skin (2 percent) (Johns and Wright 1962). However, most efforts to increase flexibility through stretching should be directed at the muscle fascia for two reasons. First, muscle and its fascia have more elastic tissue, so they are more modifiable in terms of reducing resistance to elongation. Second, because ligaments and tendons have less elasticity than fascia, it is undesirable to produce too much slack in them. Overstretching these structures may weaken the integrity of the joints. As a result, excessive flexibility may destabilize the joints and increase an athlete's risk of injury. Because the connective tissues probably play the largest role in limiting an athlete's range of motion, they must be stretched properly, such as by following the directions in part IV of this book, to develop optimal flexibility.

Bones and Joints

Ultimately, an athlete's range of motion at a joint is restricted by both the bone and the joint structure. Just as the railroad track determines the route available to the train, so the shape and contour of the joint surfaces ultimately determine the movement. Pathways are further influenced by cartilage, ligaments, tendons, and other connective tissues that frequently serve as restraining factors.

The pelvic region exemplifies the correlation between bone and joint structure and range of movement (figure 5, *a* and *b*). Some of the structural characteristics of the female pelvis that differ from the male pelvis are these:

- Bones are lighter.
- Brim is rounder.
- Cavity is shallower and more capacious.
- Outlet is larger.
- Sacrosciatic notch is wider.
- Acetabula are farther apart.
- Subpubic angle is wider.
- Sacrum is wider and more curved.

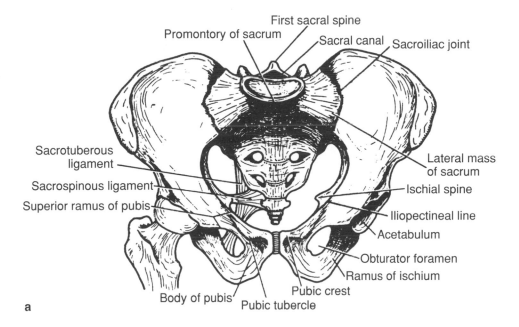

a

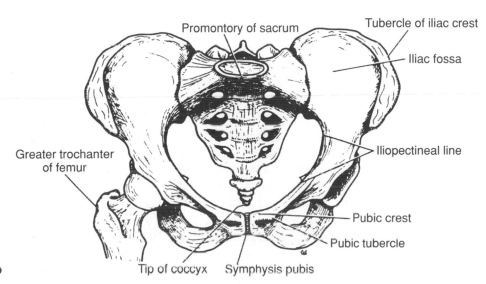

b

Figure 5 The male (*a*) and female (*b*) pelvis.

Reprinted, with permission, from R.S. Snell, 1992, *Clinical anatomy for medical students,* 4th ed. (Boston: Little, Brown), 313.

It is important for athletes and coaches to understand that the female's pelvis generally allows a greater range of flexibility than the male's. The most significant structural reasons for a female's enhanced flexibility are broader hips and a less shallow pelvic cavity (acetabulum). In particular, the less shallow pelvis permits greater joint play and hence ROM in the pelvic region.

WHAT HAPPENS WHEN YOU STRETCH?

Several types of adaptation result from proper and regular stretching. First, as stated earlier, when a muscle is suddenly stretched, the stretch reflex is initiated and the muscle being stretched contracts. However, through training, the critical point at which the stretch reflex is initiated can be "reset" to a higher level. Consequently, your muscles relax farther into the stretch. Research in the field of neurophysiology has demonstrated adaptive plasticity in the central nervous system (Wolpaw and Carp 1990). Specifically, the magnitude of the spinal stretch reflex can be uptrained (increased), downtrained (decreased), or even trained to reverse the changed response. Wolpaw and Carp's study (1990) has even substantiated the hypothesis that altered reflex activity eventually modifies the plasticity of the spinal cord neural circuits.

Second, with increased stretching over time, the number of sarcomeres is thought to increase in series. These new sarcomeres are added onto the end of the existing myofibrils. Research has substantiated that an addition of sarcomeres is responsible for an increase in muscle length (Goldspink 1968; Williams and Goldspink 1971). However, additional research is needed to substantiate that an increase in the number of sarcomeres actually results from a traditional stretching program used in an athletic setting.

Third, with increased stretching over time the fascial sheaths encasing your muscles—the epimysium, endomysium, and perimysium (refer to figure 4)—may undergo semipermanent change in length. Other tissues adapting to the stretch are the tendons, ligaments, fascia, and scar tissue.

Fourth, stretching exercises are known to increase passive range of motion and extensibility of the hamstrings. However, research has also shown that stretching exercises do not make short hamstrings less stiff. Rather, increased extensibility is attributed to an increase in stretch tolerance (Halbertsma and Göeken 1994; Halbertsma, van Bolhuis, and Göeken 1996).

Fifth, research suggests that muscle cells may control and modulate stiffness and elastic limit coordinately by selective expression of specific titin isoforms (structural variants) (Wang et al. 1991); that is, muscles that express greater titin isoforms tend to initiate tension at longer sarcomere lengths, reach their elastic limit at higher sarcomere lengths, and develop the lowest tension. Such control and modulation may be influenced by training.

Sixth, stretching is thought to stimulate the production and retention of gel-like substances called glycoaminoglycans (GAGs). The GAGs, along with water and hyaluronic acid, lubricate connective tissue fibers, maintaining a critical distance between them. This prevents the fibers from touching one another and sticking together. As a result, excessive cross-linkages are not formed (figure 6) (Akeson, Amiel, and Woo 1980).

Seventh, x-ray studies (Nikolic and Zimmermann 1968) have demonstrated that training can modify the bone and joint structure in dancers; hence, range of motion can be enhanced, and stretching is one way to do this.

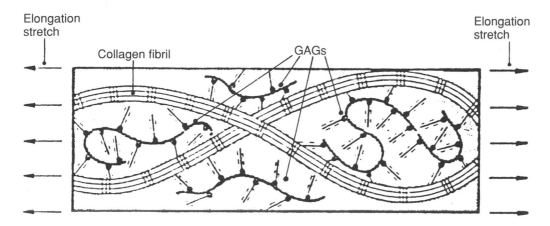

Figure 6 The action of GAGs. Stretch is applied to collagen fibrils, but the GAGs keep the fibrils separated and aligned.

Reprinted, with permission, from E.R. Myers, C.G. Armstrong, and V.C. Mow, 1984, Swelling, Pressure, and Collagen Tension. In *Connective tissue matrix*, ed. D.W.L. Hukin. (Deerfield Beach, FL: Verlag Chemie), 171.

Last, recent research suggests that mechanical stimulation (e.g., stretching or resistance training) of muscle and connective tissues may affect gene expression (Simpson et al. 1994; Sutcliffe and Davidson 1990). This, in turn, may modulate tissue variants and thus influence muscle and connective tissue extensibility.

STRETCHING TECHNIQUES

Stretching refers to the process of elongation. Stretching exercises are performed in a variety of ways, depending on your goals, abilities, and state of training. For example, a world-class gymnast or black belt in karate may perform more advanced stretches than individuals who are beginning stretching programs simply to improve their personal health and fitness. There are five basic stretching techniques: static, ballistic, passive, active, and proprioceptive.

Static Stretching

Static stretching involves stretching to the farthest point and holding the stretch. Splits are a good example of static stretching. This method of stretching is not only the safest, but also has been test proven for centuries by practitioners of hatha yoga as a means of enhancing flexibility. Other advantages are that it

- is simple to learn and easy to execute,
- requires little expenditure of energy,
- allows adequate time to reset the sensitivity of the stretch reflex,
- permits semipermanent change in length, and
- can induce muscular relaxation via firing of the GTOs if the stretch is sufficiently intense.

The major disadvantage of static stretching is its lack of specificity. During the early 1960s, the S.A.I.D. Principle, developed by Wallis and Logan (1964), put forth the idea that ideally athletes should develop their strength, endurance, and flexibility based on the principle of specific adaptation to imposed demands; that is, one should stretch at not less than 75 percent of maximum velocity through the exact plane of motion, through the exact range of motion, and at the precise joint angles used while performing skills in a specific activity. Research studies substantiate the concepts of sport specificity and the S.A.I.D. Principle. Because most activities and movements are dynamic in nature, static stretching does little to enhance coordination and does not offer optimal specificity in training. Remember, muscle has two types of receptors: The primary endings measure both velocity and muscle length, whereas the secondary endings measure length alone. Thus, dynamic stretching must be used to condition the primary endings for their desired response.

In addition, one study (Rosenbaum and Hennig 1995) suggested that it is advisable not to apply solely static stretching routines because of "a potentially impairing effect on muscle performance" (p. 489). Specifically, their research found stretching had a negative effect on active force production. A possible rationale for this negative effect may be due to mechanical characteristics changes of the damping ratio (the ability to absorb and dissipate shock loading) and mechanical stiffness (the ability to resist deformation) of soft tissues (Siff 1993a).

Ballistic and Dynamic Stretching

Ballistic stretching involves bobbing, bouncing, rebounding, and rhythmic types of movement. As mentioned earlier, in ballistic stretching, momentum is the driving force that moves the body or limb to forcibly increase the ROM. This technique is the most controversial stretching method because it can cause the most soreness and injury. Other disadvantages are that it

- fails to provide adequate time for the tissues to adapt to the stretch; and
- initiates the stretch reflex and thereby increases muscular tension, making it more difficult to stretch the connective tissues.

Based on the above disadvantages, athletes may choose to incorporate dynamic rather than ballistic stretching into their training regime. The key difference between ballistic and dynamic stretching is that the latter does not end with bouncing or jerky movements. Instead, the movements are under control. Research has demonstrated that both ballistic and dynamic stretching enhance flexibility; however, dynamic stretching develops optimum dynamic flexibility, essential for all sports. Remember, flexibility training must be velocity specific to condition and train the velocity-specific stretch receptors.

A safe ballistic (dynamic) stretching program has been developed by Zachazewski (1990). He recommends a progressive velocity flexibility program (PVFP) preceded by a warm-up. Then, over time, the athlete goes through "a series of stretching exercises in which the velocity and range of lengthening are combined and controlled on a progressive basis" (p. 228). This gradual program permits the muscle and musculotendinous junction to adapt progressively to functional ballistic movements, hence reducing the risk of injury. Zachazewski (1990; see figure 7) briefly describes the program as follows:

The athlete progresses from an environment of control to activity simulation, from slow-velocity methodical activity to high-velocity functional activity. After static-stretching, slow short end range (SSER) ballistic stretching is initiated. The athlete then progresses to slow full range stretching (SFR), fast short end range (FSER) and fast full range (FFR) stretching. Control and range are the responsibility of the athlete. No outside force is exerted by anyone else. (p. 228)

In contrast, Tom Kurz, a leading flexibility instructor, challenges the generally accepted belief that static stretching should be employed after an initial warm-up routine. He contends that "doing static stretches before a workout consisting of dynamic actions is counterproductive." Instead, he advocates using dynamic stretches first and static stretching when the major part of the workout is completed and it is time for cool-down (Kurz 1994).

Passive Stretching

Passive stretching is a technique in which you are relaxed and make no contribution to the range of motion. Instead, an external force is created by a manual or mechanical outside agent. Passive stretching is preferred when the elasticity of the muscles and connective tissues to be stretched (antagonists) restricts flexibility and for muscles or tissues undergoing rehabilitation. Among the advantages associated with passive stretching are the following:

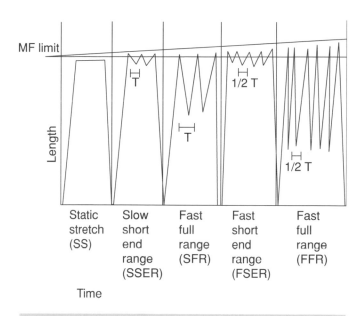

Figure 7 A progressive velocity flexibility program (PVFP). MF limit is the muscle flexibility limit of the muscle being stretched.

Reprinted, with permission, from J.E. Zachazewski, 1990, Flexibility for sports. In *Sports physical therapy*, ed. B. Sanders. (Norwalk, CT: Appleton & Lange), 234.

- It is effective when the agonist (the primary muscle responsible for the movement) is too weak to respond.
- It is effective when attempts to inhibit the tight muscles are unsuccessful.
- It is preferred when the elasticity of the muscles to be stretched (antagonists) restricts flexibility.
- It allows stretching beyond one's active range of motion.
- It provides a reserve for increasing the joint's active mobility.
- Direction, duration, and intensity can be measured when more advanced stretching machines and modalities are used in rehabilitative therapy.
- It can promote team camaraderie when athletes stretch with partners.

Athletes need to recognize several disadvantages with regard to passive stretching. First, there is greater risk of soreness and injury if a partner applies the external force incorrectly. In addition, passive stretching may initiate the stretch reflex if the stretch is too rapid. Another important disadvantage is that the likelihood of injury increases with greater differences between the ranges of active and passive flexibility (Iashvili 1983) (figure 8). But perhaps most important for the athlete, research has demonstrated that passive flexibility values have a lower correlation to the level of sport achievement than active flexibility (Iashvili 1983). The solution, then, is to develop your active flexibility also.

Active Stretching

Active stretching is accomplished using your own muscles and without any assistance from an external force. Active stretching can be divided into two major classes: free active and resistive. Free active exercise or stretch occurs when muscles produce movement without application of additional external resistance. An example of free active stretching is standing upright and slowly lifting one leg to a 100-degree angle. In resistive active exercises, the athlete uses voluntary muscle contractions to move against an applied resistance. Using the previous example, a manual resistance or weight can be applied to the leg being lifted. Active stretching is preferred when the weakness of those muscles producing the movement (agonists) restricts flexibility.

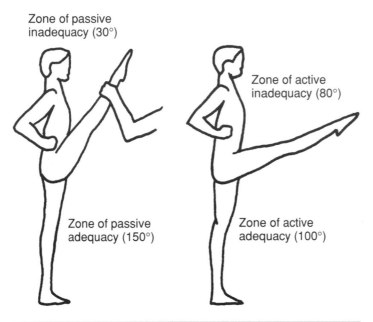

Zone of passive inadequacy (30°)

Zone of active inadequacy (80°)

Zone of passive adequacy (150°)

Zone of active adequacy (100°)

Figure 8   Flexibility zones.
Reprinted, with permission, from M.J. Alter, 1996, *Science of Flexibility*, 2nd ed. (Champaign, IL: Human Kinetics), 179.

Active stretching is vital to the athlete because it develops active (and potentially dynamic) flexibility, which in turn has been found to have a higher correlation with sport achievement than does passive flexibility (Iashvili 1983). As active stretching is most specific to a given discipline, it has the greatest potential value for the athlete. Moreover, active stretching may be easier to work into a stretching routine, as it does not require a partner or other equipment. The major disadvantages of active stretching are that it may initiate the stretch reflex and that it may be ineffective in the presence of certain dysfunctions and injuries such as severe sprains, inflammation, or fractures.

In recent years, a modified version called active-assisted stretching has become increasingly popular. With active-assisted stretching, the range of motion is completed by a partner or device (inner tube or towel) when one's limit of flexibility is reached. The advantage of this modified technique is that it can activate or strengthen the weak agonist opposing the tight muscle, help establish the pattern for coordinated motion, and allow stretching beyond one's active range of motion. Research is needed to quantify and substantiate claims of enhanced performance for athletes.

Proprioceptive Neuromuscular Facilitation

Proprioceptive neuromuscular facilitation is another broad strategy that can be implemented to improve your range of motion. A modified version of one of the PNF techniques is referred to in osteopathic medicine as a muscle energy technique. PNF was originally designed and developed as a rehabilitative physical therapy procedure. Today, several different types of PNF are being used in the arena of sports medicine. Names and descriptions of PNF techniques vary according to source; therefore, comparisons are often difficult to assess. In this text, we have adopted the terminology and description of Moore and Hutton (1980). Two of the more prevalent PNF strategies in athletic training are the contract-relax and contract-relax-agonist-contract techniques.

Contract-Relax (CR) Technique.   The contract-relax technique (also called hold-relax technique) starts with the athlete's tight muscle group (antagonist) in a lengthened position. Assume for the sake of illustration that your hamstrings are tight. The tight hamstrings are first gently stretched and gradually contract isometrically, building to a less than maximum effort for 6 to 15 seconds against a partner's resistance. As the contraction is isometric, there is no change in the muscle's length or movement of the joint. This contraction is followed by a brief period of relaxing the hamstrings. Then the partner slowly lengthens the tight muscle group (hamstrings) by passively moving the extremity through its gained range of motion (figure 9, *a* and *b*).

The rationale for the contract-relax technique is that the initial contraction of the antagonists (hamstrings) in the stretched position is thought to promote a subsequent relaxation phase of the same muscle. In part, this relaxation may be a result of the inhibitory activity from the GTOs. Still, it is

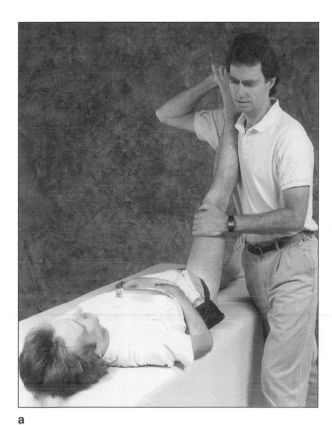
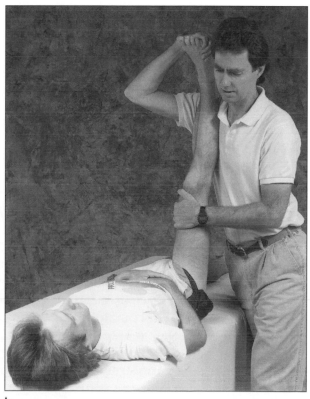

a   b

Figure 9   (*a*) Starting position of the PNF contract-relax hamstring stretch. (*b*) The stretcher actively deepens the stretch.

Reprinted, with permission, from R.E. McAtee, 1993, *Facilitated stretching*. (Champaign, IL: Human Kinetics), 14-15.

important to perform PNF relaxation techniques rapidly to achieve the desired inhibitory (relaxation) effect. Because the effect of the maximal depression lasts less than one second and 70 percent recovery occurs within five seconds, Moore and Kukulka (1991) suggest that "stretch increments should be applied immediately after the voluntary contraction, preferably within the first second and certainly by five seconds postcontraction."

Contract-Relax-Agonist-Contract (CRAC) Technique.   The contract-relax-agonist-contract technique is similar to the CR technique except that the relaxation phase is followed by an active contraction of the agonist (i.e., the antagonist of the tight muscle group, which in this instance are the quadriceps muscles). This last phase can also be assisted by the partner. Then the entire procedure is repeated.

The CRAC technique is based on the neurophysiology of reciprocal inhibition; that is, when the agonists (quadriceps) contract, the antagonists (hamstrings) relax. In addition, the CRAC method has been found to produce the greatest range of motion compared to other techniques (Moore and Hutton 1980). Another potential advantage is the facilitation of active flexibility. The major disadvantage of the CRAC technique is more discomfort and perceived pain.

Two frequently asked questions regarding the contraction phase of PNF exercises deal with its intensity and length of time. The originators of PNF and most early literature used the term *maximal* to describe the proper amount of resistance. However, many PNF instructors now consider the terms *optimal* or *appropriate* more accurate (Adler, Beckers, and Buck, 1993). This text uses *less than maximal* isometric contractions as recommended by McAtee (1993). The advantages include safety, less soreness, less tiring for the partner, and partners being able to work together despite differences in size and strength (McAtee 1993).

Length of time has been analyzed in a study comparing isometric contraction periods of zero, three, and six seconds. The research supported the hypothesis of the superiority of longer isometric contractions in active PNF groups; however, this superiority is absent from passive PNF groups (Hardy 1985). Further study of this complex issue is necessary.

PNF techniques offer a wider range of advantages and benefits than other conventional stretching methods. Most significant, PNF seems to be the most successful method for developing flexibility. The technique is also praised because it enhances active flexibility and helps establish a pattern for coordinated motion. It is also considered superior because it uses several important neurophysiological mechanisms, such as reciprocal innervation and the inverse myotatic reflex. PNF techniques are also thought to help reset the stretch reflex level or alter stretch perception (Magnusson et al. 1996). However, many of these assumptions have been challenged (Moore and Hutton 1980).

Unfortunately, PNF techniques have several disadvantages. Most important is the greater risk of injury, ranging from a pulled muscle to certain cardiovascular complications. Furthermore, the technique requires a knowledgeable and well-trained partner, which can be uneconomical in a practice session because one athlete (the partner) is neither stretching nor resting (Kurz 1994).

Stretching Aids

In addition to the techniques described above, there is another way to enhance range of motion by using specifically designed stretching machines. Stretching machines have been extensively promoted since the mid-1970s in a variety of dance, gymnastics, martial arts, and yoga magazines. These machines vary in cost and sophistication. Dependent upon design and utilization, stretching machines can facilitate the development of either active, static, or passive flexibility. Perhaps the most popular and widely promoted device is the "rack" design (figure 10).

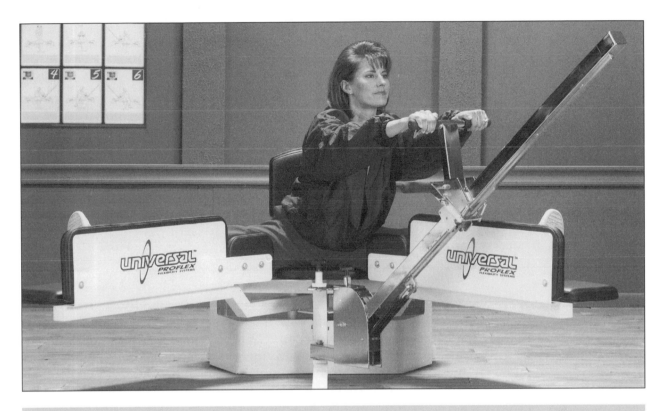

Figure 10 Universal Proflex stretching machine.
Note: The Universal Proflex is no longer available for purchase.
Photo furnished by Universal Gym Equipment, Inc., West Palm Beach, FL.

Consider a number of factors prior to purchasing any stretching device, including the safety, effectiveness, and durability of the product. Seek a knowledgeable certified athletic trainer, physical therapist, or physician to help evaluate a stretching device's safety and effectiveness. Ask the manufacturer if the device does what it claims or provides a free trial with a money-back guarantee. Also inquire how long the warranty lasts, what is necessary to get a temporary replacement, and how long it takes to get a replacement. Consider the materials and components that make up the machine. How sturdy is the device, and how will it stand up to wear and tear? Also consider the ease of operation or user friendliness of design. Does the machine require special training? Is it bulky, heavy, and large (making it difficult to store)?

WHAT CAUSES MUSCULAR SORENESS?

Athletes commonly experience discomfort, soreness, stiffness, or pain. These afflictions fall into two general categories: those that occur during and immediately

KNOWING A JOINT'S MAXIMUM SUSTAINABLE ACTIVE AND PASSIVE FLEXIBILITY

It is prudent to explain why coaches and athletes need to understand the importance of (1) developing both passive and active flexibility and (2) having quantified data on the limits of a joint's allowable active and passive range of motion. "By knowing the amount of reserve (the high rating of passive mobility) and the actual (passive and active) mobility in joints, one can determine the amount of potential increase" (Karmenov 1990). Calculate the potential increase of active flexibility by subtracting the measure of active flexibility from the measure of passive flexibility. This difference is the zone of active inadequacy. For example, given the amount of passive adequacy (flexibility) is 150 degrees, and the active adequacy (flexibility) is 100 degrees, then the potential increase in active flexibility is 50 degrees. Thus, the greater zone of active inadequacy, the greater is the potential to increase active flexibility. It is important to note, however, that there is also an increased likelihood of injury with greater differences between the ranges of active and passive flexibility (Iashvili 1983).

Determine the potential increase in passive adequacy (flexibility) by subtracting the passive adequacy from the amount of reserve mobility, i.e., the high rating of passive mobility. This difference is the zone of passive inadequacy (see figure 8). For example, assume that elite acrobats or gymnasts should possess 180 degrees of hip flexion with the legs kept straight. (This high rating of passive mobility would be determined from standardized test data that establish set norms for related age groups.) If the zone of passive adequacy is 150 degrees, then the potential increase in passive adequacy is

180 degrees − 150 degrees = 30 degrees

Such information can assist coaches and trainers in improving performance and reducing the risk of injury.

---

after the exercise (these may persist for several hours) and those that usually do not appear until 24 to 48 hours later. This muscle soreness can also occur as a result of stretching. Therefore, athletes and coaches need to understand what causes soreness to develop and implement strategies to eliminate or minimize its occurrence. Currently, there are four basic hypotheses that attempt to explain the nature of muscular soreness. Although these will be discussed separately, they can occur together. There also may be other causes of muscular soreness.

Torn or Damaged Tissue

This hypothesis states that soreness results from the microscopic tearing of muscle fibers or connective tissues (figure 11, *a* and *b*). More recently, this has been expanded into the connective tissue damage hypothesis, which suggests that the soreness is due to irritation or damage of connective tissue—usually a result of exercises or training that use eccentric contractions (for instance, the elongation or stretching of a muscle while it is contracting under resistance). Plyometrics is an example of a training technique that uses eccentric contractions.

Metabolic Accumulation, Pressure, and Swelling

This hypothesis emphasizes the accumulation of muscle metabolic by-products, leading to retained excess water (edema). In turn, the pressure on the athlete's sensory nerves creates the pain. An analogy is to compare muscle with a water balloon stuffed inside a nylon stocking. The increased volume of fluid produces passive tension throughout the stocking, resulting in pain, swelling, and stiffness. Although several researchers believe this theory is questionable, if not unlikely, it has yet to be disproved.

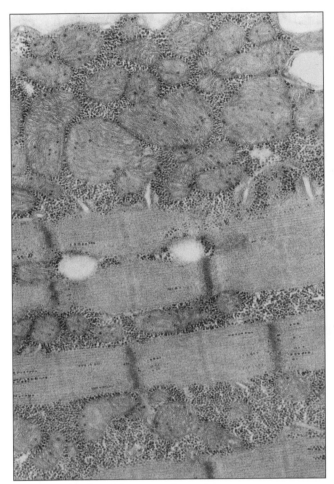
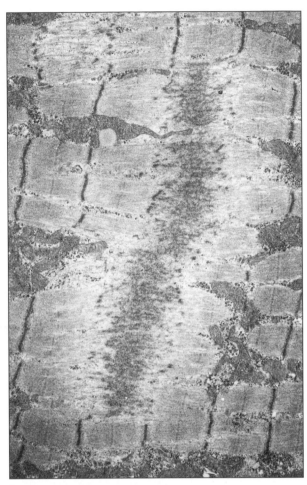

a

b

Figure 11 (*a*) An electron micrograph showing normal arrangement of the actin and myosin filaments and Z-disk configuration in the muscle of a runner before a marathon. (*b*) A muscle sample taken immediately after a marathon race shows a damaged sarcomere.

Reprinted, with permission, from J.H. Wilmore and D.L. Costill, 1994, *Physiology of sport*. (Champaign, IL: Human Kinetics), 79.

Lactic Acid Hypothesis

Lactic acid is a waste by-product of metabolism and can only form in the absence of oxygen. Therefore, lactic acid accumulates only when there is insufficient blood supply to the muscles. Consequently, lactic acid must not be a factor in pain following passive exercise and most static stretching programs.

Muscle Spasms

The localized spasm of motor units hypothesis developed by de Vries (1961, 1966) is intended to explain delayed localized soreness. By this hypothesis, exercise above a minimal level causes decreased blood flow to the muscle, or ischemia, which in turn causes pain that results in a protective reflex tonic muscle contraction. The tonic contraction brings about more ischemia, and a vicious cycle is born. Here, too, researchers have been unable to substantiate the findings of de Vries. Localized spasms may indeed be a source of localized pain; however, the proposal that the initial cause is due to decreased blood flow to the muscle should not be a factor in pain following passive and static stretching exercises incorporated in athletic programs.

Some degree of soreness is often experienced by those who have not previously exercised or stretched—this is the penalty for having been inactive. The best ways to minimize the risk of soreness associated with stretching are as follows:

1. Precede stretching with a sufficient warm-up period.
2. Implement a progressive velocity flexibility program.
3. Use correct technique.
4. Do not neglect to develop other major components of fitness: agility, balance, endurance, strength, power, and speed.

Nonetheless, even well-trained athletes who work out at higher than usual levels of difficulty can also become sore or injured.

APPROPRIATE INJURY MANAGEMENT

If muscle soreness or an injury occurs, determine to the best of your knowledge the extent of the damage. As a general rule, rest, apply ice and pressure, and elevate the injured part of the body, then seek appropriate medical care. The sooner an injury is treated, the earlier rehabilitation can begin and the faster recovery will be.

HOW AGING AFFECTS FLEXIBILITY

Flexibility can be developed at any age, given the appropriate training; however, the rate of development may not be the same at every age for all athletes. Generally, research indicates that small children are quite supple, and that during the school years flexibility decreases until about puberty, then increases throughout adolescence. After adolescence, however, flexibility tends to level off and then decrease. Although flexibility decreases with age, the loss appears to be minimized in those who remain active. Research has found that maturational age as measured by sexual maturity, rather than by chronological age, was better correlated with strength and flexibility in the lower extremity. However, many parents, coaches, and adolescent athletes fail "to consider developmental variation [which] often leads to inappropriate performance expectations and an unsatisfactory sports experience" (Pratt 1989).

A primary factor responsible for flexibility decreasing with age is certain changes in the connective tissues of the body. Interestingly, it has been suggested that exercise delays the loss of flexibility due to dehydration within the connective tissues. This is based on the notion that stretching stimulates the production or retention of lubricants between the connective tissue fibers, thus preventing adhesions. Other physical changes that occur with aging and affect flexibility include

- increased calcium deposits,
- increased dehydration in connective tissues,
- increased adhesions and cross-links in the connective tissues,
- an actual change in the chemical structure of the tissues, and
- the replacement of muscle fibers with fatty and fibrous (collagen) fibers.

ADDING A STRETCHING PROGRAM TO YOUR WORKOUT

A flexibility training program is a planned, deliberate, and regular program of exercises that can permanently and progressively increase the usable range of motion of a joint or set of joints over time (Aten and Knight 1978). In the arena of athletics, training in general is a multisided process to influence the development of an athlete and ensure the necessary level of preparation. Stretching exercises comprise just one essential component of an athlete's total training program.

Warming Up

A warm-up consisting of exercises performed immediately before an activity to increase circulation and heart rate is an essential part of a good conditioning program. Warm-up exercises provide an athlete with time to adjust from rest to exercise. These exercises are designed to improve performance and reduce the chance of injury by preparing the athlete mentally as well as physically for his or her sport. Physiologically, a warm-up elevates body temperature and increases blood flow.

Stretching is often incorrectly considered synonymous with warm-up because it is commonly done during the warm-up portion of a training program. In addition, static and passive stretching exercises do virtually nothing to increase core or peripheral temperatures and blood flow; hence, these stretching techniques do not serve as a warm-up. In fact, stretching should always be preceded by a warm-up because the elevated tissue temperature enhances connective tissue and muscular extension, thereby reducing the risk of injury from stretching.

Warm-up routines are typically classified into three categories. A passive warm-up involves raising the body temperature by some external means such as heating pads and hot showers. A general warm-up is probably the most commonly used technique. It employs various movements not directly related to those employed in the activity itself. These include joint rotations and gentle twisting and bending movements. This is usually followed by light calisthenics, brisk walking, jogging, or jumping rope. Here the goal is to increase muscle blood flow and raise core body temperature. A formal or specific warm-up includes movements that either mimic or are employed in the actual activity, performed at a reduced level of intensity.

The intensity and duration of a warm-up must be suited to the athlete's physical capabilities and adjusted to the existing conditions. Generally, an athlete's warm-up should be intense enough to increase body temperature and cause some sweating but not so intense as to cause fatigue. A warm-up should be more intense in cold weather.

BENEFITS OF A GOOD WARM-UP

- Increase in body and tissue temperature
- Increase of blood flow through the active muscles
- Increase in heart rate, which prepares the cardiovascular system for work
- Increase in the rate of energy release in the body (the metabolic rate)
- Increase in the exchange of oxygen from hemoglobin
- Increase in speed at which nerve impulses travel, facilitating body movements
- Increase in reciprocal innervation efficiency (allowing muscles to contract and relax faster and more efficiently)
- Decrease in muscular tension
- Enhanced ability of connective tissue to elongate
- Help in preparing the athlete psychologically

Duration, Frequency, Timing, and Intensity

There is much debate and little consensus about recommendations for duration, frequency, timing, and intensity of flexibility training (Alter 1996). Consider several important factors when designing a flexibility training program. Perhaps most important, the athlete or coach must identify the purpose of the flexibility training session. Specifically, is the purpose of the program development, maintenance, or rehabilitation of flexibility?

Ideally, a training program should be individually tailored to meet the needs of the athlete; however, many athletes train in a group or team flexibility program. This team-centered program is advantageous because it guarantees at least a minimal amount of stretching and fosters camaraderie and team spirit. However, in such cases, it is still essential that each individual athlete be properly instructed to concentrate on specific areas that need additional stretching on the athlete's own time. Let's briefly review what is commonly recommended for most healthy individuals.

Most programs recommend holding each stretch for 6 to 30 seconds. The problem with holding stretches for longer than 30 seconds is that warm-up and stretching programs in combination might last longer than many workouts. Furthermore, one study found that 30 seconds of static stretching of the hamstring muscles was as effective as the longer duration of 1 minute (Bandy and Irion 1994). This text recommends two to three repetitions of each stretch held for 10 seconds or one repetition of each stretch held for 20 to 30 seconds. The reasoning is simple: Lack of flexibility is primarily due to connective tissue whose permanent or plastic deformation is most favored by low-force, long-duration stretching (Sapega et al. 1981). If there is not enough time to optimally stretch during regular workout sessions, athletes must plan to stretch on their own time.

In fact, empirical evidence would probably reveal that the most significant contributing factor to dancer, gymnast, or martial artist improving his or her flexibility takes place when the individual stretches during his or her own time! Furthermore, it is tempting to speculate that as a consequence there is an increase in the passive flexibility reserve. In turn, this increased passive flexibility reserve increases one's potential for active flexibility. Consequently, it may be that passive or static flexibility is developed primarily on one's own, at home, whereas active or functional flexibility is developed in the dance studio, gym, or dojo where the passive flexibility is transformed into finely coordinated and skilled movement. Serious athletes must develop both their passive flexibility and active flexibility.

As training progresses, increase the number of successive repetitions for each routine. In addition, incorporate dynamic stretching performed in series, with a gradual increase in range of motion. The number of repetitions in series usually ranges from 8 to 12, but well-trained athletes may perform as many as 40 or more repetitions with maximum amplitude (Matveyev 1981). Some experts recommend three to six sets of 10 to 15 repetitions (Costill, Maglischo, and Richardson 1992). Keep in mind that fatigue and the consequent reduction in amplitude is a sign to stop (Harre 1982). If your muscles begin to quiver and vibrate, pain persists, or range of motion decreases, you have stretched too much. As a general rule, nonathletes should stretch at least once a day, three to five days per week, to maintain flexibility. Depending on their sport, dedicated and serious athletes may require two to three stretching sessions per day for six or seven days per week.

When within a workout session should stretching exercises be done? Research refutes that specific placement of stretching exercises within a workout session makes a difference in increasing range of motion (Cornelius, Hagemann, and Jackson 1988). However, Sapega et al. (1981) recommend incorporating stretching immediately after the main part of a workout and cool-down period because tissue temperatures are highest, making stretching both safer and more productive.

Another question then arises: How intense should a stretch be to develop flexibility? Because intensity is based on subjective factors (tension, discomfort, pain), there is no way for coaches or trainers to determine this level for their athletes; the intensity of the stretch must be up to the athlete. In general, stretch to the point of tension but not pain. For athletes who are undergoing rehabilitation and have healing tissues, the point before pain is reached may be sufficient to rupture already weakened tissues. Remember, the best advice is to use common sense: Train, don't strain.

Improving and retaining flexibility depend on numerous variables, including genetic factors, age, and the state of training. Thus, your muscles' responses to regular stretching are a function of these factors and are dependent on which muscle group you stretch. Generally, for healthy individuals, the longer, more frequently, and more intensely you stretch, the faster and more significant your improvement in flexibility will be. If you are healthy, uninjured, and just starting a stretching program, you may feel increased muscle tightness and some muscle soreness the first week. But as your body adapts to regular stretching, you'll begin to see increases in your flexibility. Likewise, once you stop your stretching program, the flexibility gains will be lost over time.

Cooling Down

Cooling down is defined as performing a group of light exercises immediately after an activity to provide the body with a period of adjustment from exercise to rest. The cool-down period is valuable for athletes who want to maintain or enhance their flexibility. As tissue temperatures rise, stiffness decreases and extensibility increases. Because tissue temperatures will be highest immediately after a workout and during the cool-down phase, stretching is thought to be both safer and more productive.

Strength Training and Flexibility

Strength training is a vital component for athletes, although misconceptions exist regarding the relationship between strength training and flexibility (Todd 1985). Research demonstrates that weight training does not decrease flexibility and in some instances actually improves it (Wilmore et al. 1978). With proper training that is technically correct, an athlete can improve both overall strength and flexibility.

A common belief is that strength training significantly increases range of motion if: (1) stretching exercises are included in the training program, (2) both the agonist and antagonist muscle groups are trained, (3) the entire muscle or muscle group is worked through its full range of motion, and (4) there is a gradual emphasis on accentuating the negative phase of work. Negative work or eccentric contractions take place when a muscle is stretched (elongated) while it is contracting. This eccentric contraction is associated with the lowering phase of a resistance exercise. Unfortunately, eccentric training is also associated with a greater risk of muscle soreness.

THE CONTROVERSY ABOUT STRETCHING

Although stretching exercises are thought to prevent injury and improve performance in a number of sports, stretching exercises should *not* be considered a panacea. For some athletes, excessive flexibility may destabilize joints and may actually *increase* the likelihood of ligament injury and joint separation or dislocation. Another argument is that stretching may lead to joint hypermobility. Hypermobility is said to be present when the joints are unduly lax and the range of motion is in excess of the accepted norm in most of the joints. In turn, hypermobility may be a factor in decreased positional sense (proprioceptive acuity), which may increase the risk of acute or chronic injury. Some experts also feel that excessively loose joints may lead to premature development of osteoarthritis in athletes.

What, then, are the precautions for stretching, and when is it considered inadvisable? The most commonly cited precautions are listed below.

Don't stretch an area in question if

- a bone blocks motion;
- you recently fractured a bone;
- you suspect or know of an acute inflammatory or infectious process in or around a joint;
- you have osteoporosis;
- you experience sharp, acute pain with joint movement or muscle elongation;
- you've had a recent sprain or strain;
- your joint lacks stability;
- you suffer from certain vascular or skin diseases; or
- you experience a loss of function or decrease in range of motion.

These precautions are matters of professional medical opinion, not established fact. If you have doubts or questions about whether a stretch is right for you, consult a qualified physical therapist, athletic trainer, or medical professional.

ADVANCED STRETCHES

Virtually every stretch presents some risk. The possibility of an injury depends on numerous variables, including an athlete's state of training, age, previous injuries, structural abnormalities, fatigue, and technique. So should you incorporate advanced or "controversial" stretches into your program? According to Harold B. Falls, PhD, professor of biomedical science at Southwest Missouri State University and an editorial board member of *The Physician and Sportsmedicine:* "Everything depends on the individual. There are some exercises some people can't do, and there are others that some people can do" (Lubell 1989). Mel Siff (1993b), PhD and editor of *The International Fitness Scientist* (South Africa) agrees: "There is generally no such thing as an unsafe stretch or exercise: only an unsafe way of executing any movement for a specific individual at a specific time" (p. 128).

The stretches listed below are rated "advanced." By this rating, I mean they may be too advanced or dangerous for inactive and moderately active individuals and even for some serious or elite athletes as well. These stretches are highlighted here because, although they may not be safe for everyone, they are considered essential for dance, diving, figure skating, gymnastics, martial arts, wrestling, and yoga. In these disciplines, certain advanced stretches cannot be avoided. But if you incorporate these exercises into your training program, take the appropriate preventive measures to reduce risk of injury. In general, perform these stretches as you would any other stretch in this book: slowly, deliberately, and precisely.

The Plough

The plough (stretch 236) places excessive strain on the lower back and disks and is potentially dangerous for those with low back problems. This stretch can also create a strong stretching force on the neck. Another problem with the plough is that it stretches a region frequently flexed from faulty posture and the exercise reinforces the faulty posture. Last, it compresses the lungs and heart and interferes with breathing if there is an excessive deposit of fat around the abdominal region. However, the plough is essential for those involved in judo, wrestling, some martial arts, and yoga. The easiest way to reduce the risk of injury is to learn the exercise correctly in sequential stages.

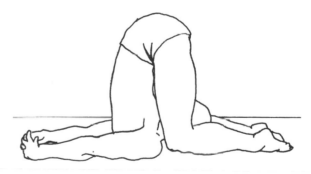

Traditional Hurdler's Stretch

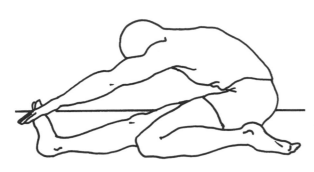

The traditional hurdler's stretch is designed to stretch the hamstrings along with the lower back muscles and related soft tissues. It also stretches the medial ligaments of the knee. For some individuals, this stretch promotes knee instability and twists and compresses the kneecap, which can cause the kneecap to side-slip. This stretch is commonly recommended for improving performance and preventing or rehabilitating injuries. The easiest way to reduce the risk of injury is to have the flexed leg positioned so that the outer side of the thigh and calf can rest on the floor, with the heel against the inner side of the opposite thigh.

Deep Knee Bend

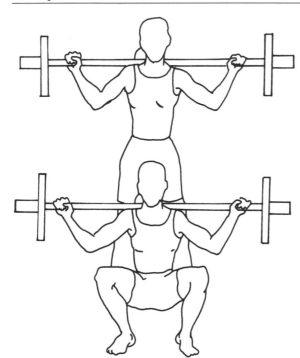

The deep knee bend (stretch 40), lunge, or squat (with or without weights) can endanger the lateral ligaments of the knee, compress the kneecap, and pinch and damage the cartilage in the knee. This stretch is a basic component of numerous skills in baseball, dance, gymnastics, handball, weight lifting, and wrestling. Minimize the degree of risk by reducing the velocity and depth of the descent and maintaining the knees over the long axis of the foot.

Standing Torso Twist

The standing torso twist (with or without weights; stretch 225) can strain the ligaments of the knee and incorporate momentum that often exceeds the absorbing capacity of the tissues being stretched. This exercise is used in many disciplines, including baseball, discus, golf, tennis, and the javelin throw. Risk-reduction strategies include placing the hands on the hips, sitting in a chair, or slightly flexing the knees when standing.

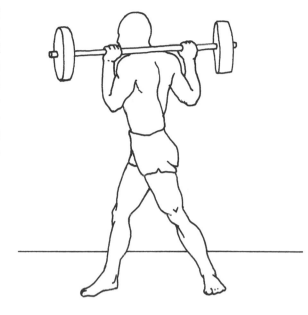

Straight-Leg Stand and Toe Touch

The straight-leg stand and toe touch (straddle or nonstraddle; stretch 75) stresses the medial aspect of the knees, forces the knee to hyperextend, places greater pressure on the lumbar spine, and can result in permanent deformity, both as loose and knock-knees. This exercise is essential in several sports and disciplines such as 3- and 10-meter diving, gymnastics, power lifting, weight lifting, and yoga. Minimize the risk of injury by avoiding ballistic movements or initiating the stretch from a squatting position.

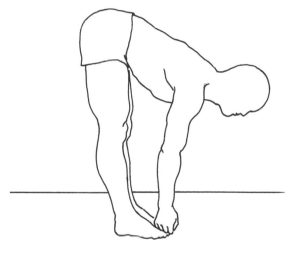

Bridge

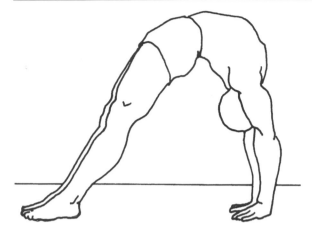

The bridge (stretch 187) squeezes the spinal disks and pinches the nerve fibers. In addition, there is concern that repetitive bridging can cause spondylolysis or low back pain. The rationale for incorporating a bridge in a training program is that it is a required skill in many disciplines such as acrobatics, gymnastics, judo, and wrestling. Risk-reduction strategies include proper sequential learning through lead-up drills and exercises, using optimal technique, and the assistance of a knowledgeable spotter.

Inversion

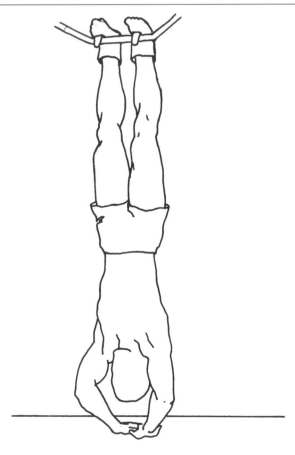

Inversion (stretch 206) raises blood pressure, may rupture blood vessels—especially in the eyes, and may injure those with spinal instability. Inversion exercises have been hypothesized to relieve or prevent low back pain, hence they are used in rehabilitation.

PART II

ALL-STAR STRETCHES

Athletes and coaches are confronted with the challenge of managing their workout time optimally. In addition, there is the dilemma of selecting a few from hundreds of potential exercises. To guarantee that a minimal level of stretching is achieved in order to optimize performance and reduce the risk of injury, I identify 12 "All-Star" stretches to serve as a series of fundamental stretches. What makes these exercises "All-Stars"? They cover the major muscle groups and regions of the body; they can be easily performed individually by healthy athletes in most disciplines; and they require just 10 to 15 minutes to perform.

12 ALL-STAR STRETCHES

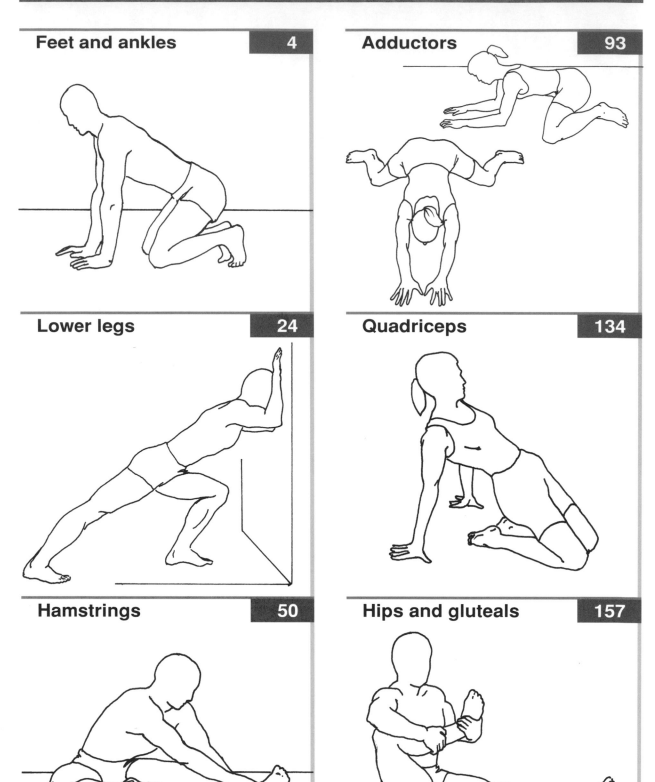

Feet and ankles	**4**	
Adductors	**93**	
Lower legs	**24**	
Quadriceps	**134**	
Hamstrings	**50**	
Hips and gluteals	**157**	

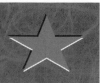
Lower torso | 197

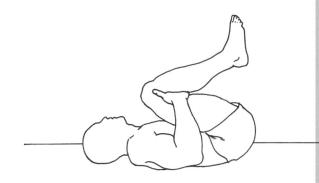

Pectorals | 250

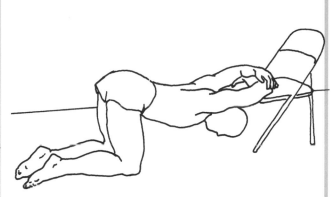

Upper back | 227

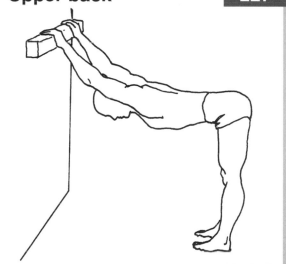

Shoulders | 280

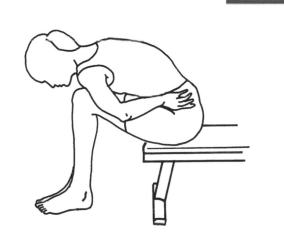

Neck | 243

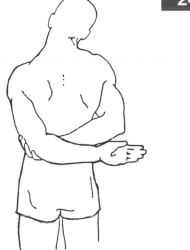

Arms and wrists | 298

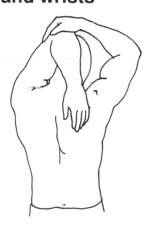

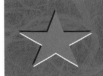
Depending upon your chosen sport, you may require more than is offered by the 12 "All-Star" Stretches. For such athletes, the 12 "All-Star" stretches may be too few in number, fail to target a specific muscle group or region, and lack sufficient intensity. Therefore, 28 muscle groups and regions have been identified with accompanying exercises that will provide the athlete with stretching exercises that are more fine-tuned and of greater intensity, yet not requiring contortionistic ranges of motion. Furthermore, all of these exercises can be performed individually with equipment found in most gyms.

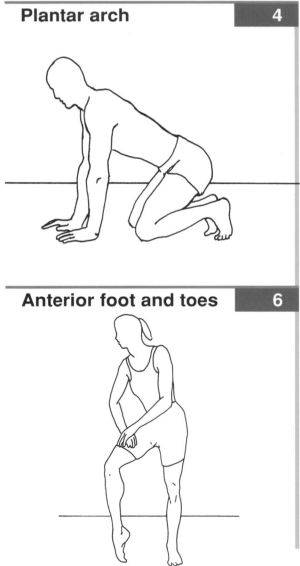

| Plantar arch | 4 |

| Anterior foot and toes | 6 |

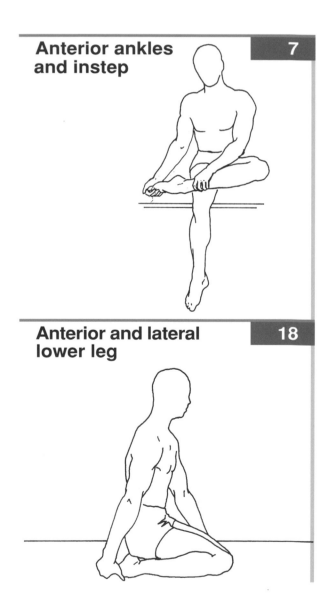

| Anterior ankles and instep | 7 |

| Anterior and lateral lower leg | 18 |

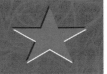

Achilles tendon and posterior lower leg | 21

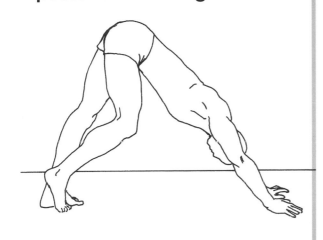

Adductors | 93

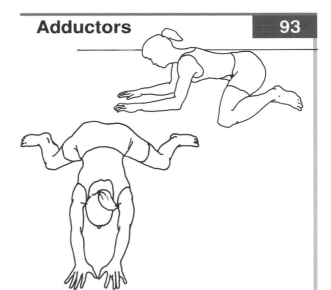

Behind the knees | 47

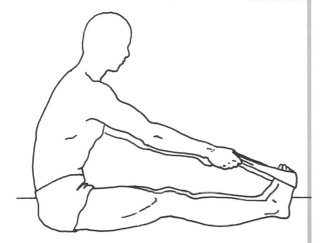

Quadriceps | 126

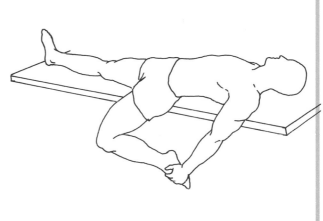

Hamstrings | 51

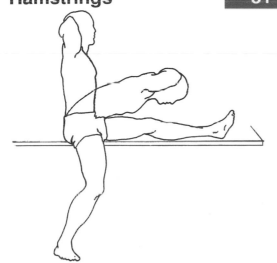

Hips and gluteals flexors | 162

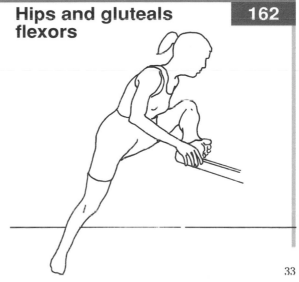

28 MAXIMAL
ISOLATION ALL-STARS
(continued)

Abdominals 180

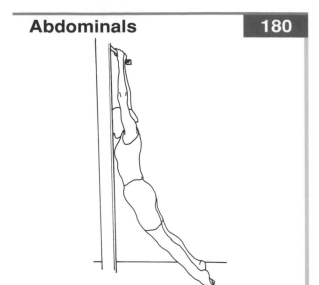

Upper back 227

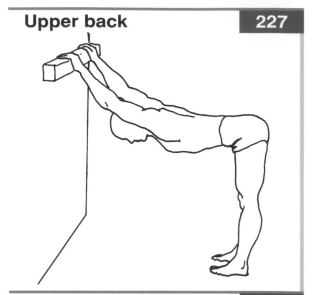

Lower back 204

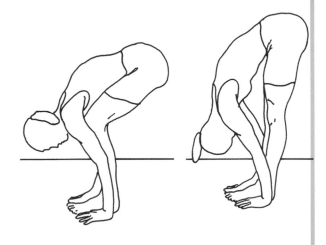

Posterior neck 240

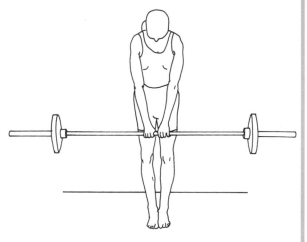

Lateral torso 215

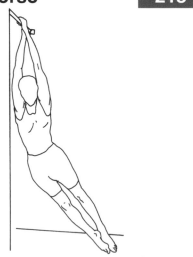

Lateral neck 244

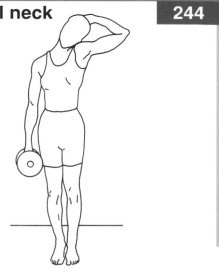

Anterior neck `245`	**Medial shoulder** `268`

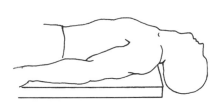

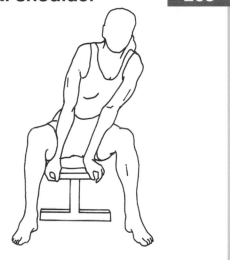

Pectorals `250`	**Lateral shoulder** `269`

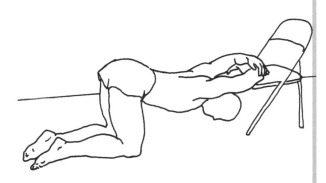

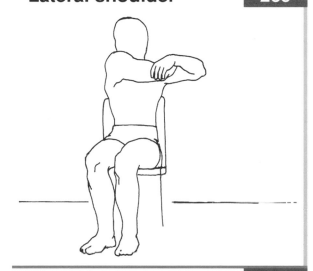

Anterior shoulder `261`	**Shoulder internal rotators (anterior)** `272`

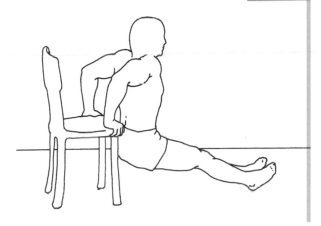

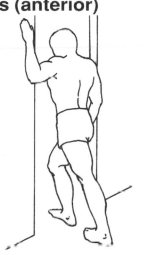

35

Shoulder external rotators (posterior) | 280

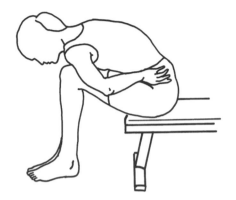

Shoulder extensors | 293

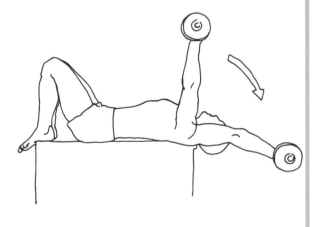

Biceps brachii | 295

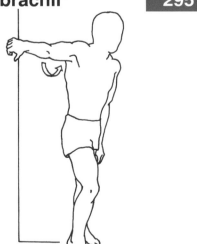

Triceps brachii | 299

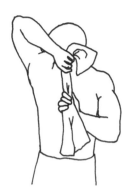

Wrist extensors | 306

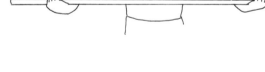

Wrist flexors | 310

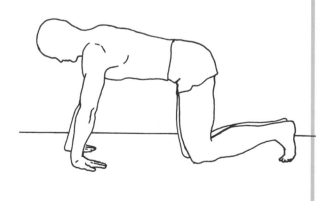

PART III

STRETCHING ROUTINES FOR SPECIFIC SPORTS

Ideally, stretching routines should be tailored to the needs and requisites of your sport. The sport-specific stretching tables (covering 41 total sports) in this section suggest routines to stretch your entire body. To stretch all 12 body regions in each table in 15 minutes, do two to three repetitions of each stretch held for 10 seconds or one repetition of each stretch held for 10 to 30 seconds. Where appropriate, repeat the stretch on the other side of the body. Each exercise in the table is ordered according to its order of appearance in part IV.

Additionally, I have highlighted and illustrated the 12 best stretches for each sport, and beneath each figure is the number that coincides with the stretch. These best stretches were determined by culling information from a variety of books and journals, from empirical evidence, and from personal experience. The stretch number helps you find the description and instructions for the stretch in part IV. If you find these best stretches either too easy or too difficult, simply substitute another that meets your needs for the same muscle group or region to come up with your own best list. You may also wish to adapt static stretches into either active, dynamic, or PNF stretches, or vice versa. The easiest way to develop your own sport-specific stretching routine is to ask questions of your coach or experiment using the stretches presented in this book.

If you are a serious athlete, the 15 minutes spent on stretching may be the most important minutes of your practice or performance session. Practical, everyday experience substantiates that flexibility enhances and optimizes the learning, practice, and performance of many skilled movements. Furthermore, proper stretching exercises may decrease the incidence, intensity, or duration of musculotendinous and joint injury.

ARCHERY

BODY PART	STRETCH NUMBER	BEST	
Feet and ankles	1, 5, 10	1	
Lower legs	16, 19, 24, 27, 28, 42	42	
Hamstrings	50, 52, 53	52	
Adductors	83, 84, 86, 88	84	
Quadriceps	119-121, 123	121	
Hips and gluteals	138, 147, 152, 155	152	
Lower torso	181, 192, 195, 197	195	
Upper back	227, 229, 230	229	
Neck	231, 242, 243, 246	231	
Pectorals	249-253, 255, 256	252	
Shoulders	259, 269, 271, 275, 276, 278	259	
Arms and wrists	295, 299, 300, 308	300	

BASEBALL, SOFTBALL, AND CRICKET
for general field players

BODY PART	STRETCH NUMBER	BEST	
Feet and ankles	2, 4, 5, 7	5	
Lower legs	16, 18, 21, 23, 26, 31, 42	21	
Hamstrings	50, 53, 63, 65	53	
Adductors	87, 91, 92, 97, 108, 111	91	
Quadriceps	119-121, 124, 131	122	
Hips and gluteals	136-138, 143, 151, 152, 157, 161, 162	161	
Lower torso	182, 192, 197, 213, 214, 222, 223	182	
Upper back	227, 229, 230	227	
Neck	231, 235, 241, 243, 246	231	
Pectorals	248, 250, 253, 255, 256	253	
Shoulders	258, 269-271, 273-276, 280	280	
Arms and wrists	295, 298, 300, 304-306, 308-310	295	

BASEBALL, SOFTBALL, AND CRICKET
for pitchers (baseball and softball) and bowlers

BODY PART	STRETCH NUMBER	BEST	
Feet and ankles	2, 3, 5, 7	7	
Lower legs	12, 23, 29	23	
Hamstrings	50, 53, 63, 65, 72	50	
Adductors	87, 88, 93, 94, 95, 100, 105	93	
Quadriceps	121, 123, 125, 126	121	
Hips and gluteals	137, 138, 151, 155, 158	155	
Lower torso	195, 202, 208, 214, 215	195	
Upper back	227, 229, 230	227	
Neck	231, 242, 243	231	
Pectorals	250, 253-256	253	
Shoulders	259, 267, 269, 271, 272, 276, 278, 280, 284, 293	280	
Arms and wrists	295, 298-300, 304, 306-311	295	

BASKETBALL

BODY PART	STRETCH NUMBER	BEST	
Feet and ankles	1, 3, 4, 5, 7, 10	3	
Lower legs	16, 18, 21, 23, 26, 28, 29, 31, 42	21	
Hamstrings	50-53, 65	51	
Adductors	83, 87, 93, 104	87	
Quadriceps	119, 120, 121, 131	121	
Hips and gluteals	136-138, 150-152, 156, 157, 172	157	
Lower torso	181, 195, 198, 213, 214	181	
Upper back	227, 229	227	
Neck	231, 235, 241, 243, 246	231	
Pectorals	248, 250, 255	250	
Shoulders	258, 259, 269, 271, 285	269	
Arms and wrists	295, 298-300, 305, 306, 308-310	310	

BOWLING

BODY PART	STRETCH NUMBER	BEST	
Feet and ankles	2, 3, 6, 10	3	
Lower legs	16, 18, 20, 29-31, 42	29	
Hamstrings	50, 53, 54, 65, 69	53	
Adductors	82-84, 91, 94, 95, 105, 117	82	
Quadriceps	119-121, 123, 134	121	
Hips and gluteals	136-138, 152, 154, 155, 157, 172	138	
Lower torso	181, 182, 194, 195, 207, 213	213	
Upper back	226, 227	227	
Neck	231, 239, 240, 242-244, 246	242	
Pectorals	249, 250	249	
Shoulders	258, 259, 269, 271, 280, 285	259	
Arms and wrists	295, 296, 298-300, 304, 306, 308-311	308	

CROSS-COUNTRY SKIING

BODY PART	STRETCH NUMBER	BEST	
Feet and ankles	2, 3, 7, 8, 10	8	
Lower legs	18, 19, 21, 23, 29, 41	19	
Hamstrings	50, 53, 65, 69, 70	53	
Adductors	88, 91, 94-96, 105, 108, 117	94	
Quadriceps	119-121, 132	121	
Hips and gluteals	152, 155, 166, 170, 172, 174	155	
Lower torso	183, 197, 213, 223-225	213	
Upper back	227, 229	227	
Neck	231, 232, 239, 240, 243, 244, 246	232	
Pectorals	250-253, 256	252	
Shoulders	259, 261, 268, 269, 276, 285, 293	269	
Arms and wrists	295, 297-300, 306, 308	298	

CYCLING AND TRIATHLON

BODY PART	STRETCH NUMBER	BEST	
Feet and ankles	4, 5, 7, 10	7	
Lower legs	16, 18, 23, 26, 28, 31, 42	31	
Hamstrings	50, 54, 65, 69-71	50	
Adductors	83, 86, 88, 91, 96, 105, 106, 117	88	
Quadriceps	119-122, 125, 131, 134	125	
Hips and gluteals	136-138, 143, 150, 152, 160-162, 174	161	
Lower torso	181, 182, 195, 197, 199, 202, 204	199	
Upper back	226, 227, 229	229	
Neck	231, 239, 240, 242, 243, 246	243	
Pectorals	248, 250, 254, 255	250	
Shoulders	258, 267, 269, 276, 278	269	
Arms and wrists	295, 298-300, 304, 305, 308-311	310	

DANCE
beginning

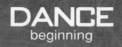

BODY PART	STRETCH NUMBER	BEST	
Feet and ankles	1-8, 10	6	
Lower legs	12, 16, 21, 23, 24, 31, 32, 34-38, 42	21	
Hamstrings	53, 55, 56, 59, 65, 66, 69	59	
Adductors	92, 93, 95, 97, 103, 105, 115	93	
Quadriceps	121, 125, 127, 134	125	
Hips and gluteals	138, 146, 157, 158, 160	160	
Lower torso	182, 194, 196, 202, 213	182	
Upper back	226, 227	227	
Neck	231, 237, 243, 246	243	
Pectorals	248, 250, 252	252	
Shoulders	257, 259, 269, 276, 277, 285	259	
Arms and wrists	295, 298-300, 305, 308-311	298	

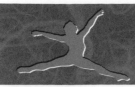

DANCE
advanced

BODY PART	STRETCH NUMBER	BEST	
Feet and ankles	1-8	8	
Lower legs	17, 18, 21, 34-38, 43	38	
Hamstrings	59, 60, 65, 66, 77	60	
Adductors	92, 93, 97, 101-103, 115	103	
Quadriceps	125, 127, 130, 135	130	
Hips and gluteals	138, 142, 145, 146, 162, 163, 174	162	
Lower torso	182, 183, 187, 202, 215	187	
Upper back	227, 229, 230	227	
Neck	231, 236, 243, 246	236	
Pectorals	250, 252-255	250	
Shoulders	259, 264, 267, 269, 279, 284, 290	279	
Arms and wrists	295, 300, 304, 308-311	300	

DIVING
3- to 10-meter

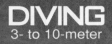

BODY PART	STRETCH NUMBER	BEST	
Feet and ankles	2, 3, 7-9	9	
Lower legs	16, 19, 23, 29, 31, 39, 40, 43, 49	29	
Hamstrings	50, 53, 55, 69, 73-77	77	
Adductors	83, 88, 93, 105, 117, 118	88	
Quadriceps	121, 125, 132, 135	125	
Hips and gluteals	138, 147, 152-157, 161, 162	155	
Lower torso	181, 182, 196, 203, 204, 214, 223-225	223	
Upper back	227, 229	227	
Neck	231, 233, 242, 246, 247	242	
Pectorals	248, 250, 252, 255	250	
Shoulders	257, 267, 269, 271, 279, 285, 286, 290	269	
Arms and wrists	295, 298-301, 304, 308	299	

47

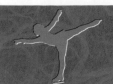

FIGURE SKATING

BODY PART	STRETCH NUMBER	BEST	
Feet and ankles	1-3, 7, 8, 10	7	
Lower legs	11, 20, 21, 24, 25, 31, 32, 39, 40	20	
Hamstrings	55, 56, 59, 60, 62, 65, 66, 77	59	
Adductors	88, 89, 93-95, 97, 101, 103, 105, 111, 117, 118	93	
Quadriceps	121, 126, 127, 128	126	
Hips and gluteals	137-139, 142, 145, 155, 161, 162, 174	162	
Lower torso	182-184, 188, 189, 197, 213, 223, 225	183	
Upper back	227, 229, 230	227	
Neck	231, 232, 237, 242, 243, 246	243	
Pectorals	250, 252, 255	250	
Shoulders	259, 269, 271, 278-280, 285, 290	269	
Arms and wrists	295, 296, 298-300, 304, 308, 309	299	

FOOTBALL
offensive line and defensive line

BODY PART	STRETCH NUMBER	BEST	
Feet and ankles	2, 3, 4, 7, 10	3	
Lower legs	16, 20, 23, 28, 31, 39-41	31	
Hamstrings	50, 52, 54, 63, 80, 81	50	
Adductors	82, 83, 88, 91, 117	91	
Quadriceps	119-121, 134	121	
Hips and gluteals	136, 137, 149, 152, 155, 157	155	
Lower torso	181, 195, 197, 210, 224, 225	197	
Upper back	227, 229	229	
Neck	231, 233, 243, 246	243	
Pectorals	248, 250, 252	252	
Shoulders	261, 269, 276, 285	269	
Arms and wrists	294, 296, 298, 304, 309, 310	298	

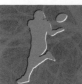

FOOTBALL
defensive backs and receivers

BODY PART	STRETCH NUMBER	BEST	
Feet and ankles	3, 4, 7	4	
Lower legs	12, 18, 21, 26, 32, 39, 46	21	
Hamstrings	50, 53, 55, 65, 81	53	
Adductors	88, 92, 93, 94, 117, 118	93	
Quadriceps	125, 127, 132, 135	135	
Hips and gluteals	138, 150, 152, 157, 161, 170	161	
Lower torso	181, 196, 197, 204, 213, 225	197	
Upper back	227, 229	227	
Neck	231, 233, 235, 243, 247	231	
Pectorals	250, 252, 255	252	
Shoulders	259, 268, 269, 271, 276, 285	269	
Arms and wrists	294, 299, 304, 308, 309	299	

GOLF

BODY PART	STRETCH NUMBER	BEST	
Feet and ankles	2, 3, 5, 7, 8	2	
Lower legs	19, 23, 28, 31, 41	28	
Hamstrings	50, 53, 54, 65	50	
Adductors	82-84, 88, 92, 105	82	
Quadriceps	121, 122, 134	121	
Hips and gluteals	137, 138, 147, 148, 152, 155, 157	155	
Lower torso	180-183, 194, 197, 208, 213, 223, 224	213	
Upper back	226, 227, 229	229	
Neck	231, 232, 240, 243, 246	243	
Pectorals	248, 249, 251, 255	251	
Shoulders	259, 268, 269, 272, 276, 280, 285	280	
Arms and wrists	295, 299, 304, 306, 308, 309	306	

GYMNASTICS

BODY PART	STRETCH NUMBER	BEST	
Feet and ankles	1, 3, 5, 8, 10	8	
Lower legs	16, 18, 21, 29, 32, 39	32	
Hamstrings	56, 59, 60, 66, 75-77	59	
Adductors	88, 93, 101, 103, 115	103	
Quadriceps	122, 125, 127, 134	125	
Hips and gluteals	138, 139, 141, 142, 160, 162	138	
Lower torso	187, 190, 191, 214, 216	187	
Upper back	226, 227	227	
Neck	231, 237, 243, 246	237	
Pectorals	250, 252, 253, 256	253	
Shoulders	262, 267, 269, 271, 284, 288, 290, 292	267	
Arms and wrists	295, 300, 306-309	309	

HIKING AND BACKPACKING

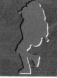

BODY PART	STRETCH NUMBER	BEST	
Feet and ankles	2, 3, 5, 7	3	
Lower legs	18-20, 29, 44, 47	18	
Hamstrings	50, 53, 54, 65, 69, 80	50	
Adductors	82, 83, 88, 94, 95, 104, 105, 117	88	
Quadriceps	119, 120, 122, 131, 133, 134	122	
Hips and gluteals	147, 155, 156, 165, 166, 169	155	
Lower torso	181, 194, 197, 210, 213, 224	210	
Upper back	226, 227, 229	227	
Neck	231, 232, 240, 243, 246	231	
Pectorals	248, 249, 250	250	
Shoulders	258, 268, 269, 276, 277, 285	269	
Arms and wrists	295, 297, 298, 304, 308	308	

ICE HOCKEY

BODY PART	STRETCH NUMBER	BEST	
Feet and ankles	1, 5, 7, 10	10	
Lower legs	13, 20, 24, 31, 32, 41	31	
Hamstrings	50, 53, 55, 63, 69	50	
Adductors	87, 91, 93, 95, 117, 118	93	
Quadriceps	119, 124, 134, 135	134	
Hips and gluteals	137, 138, 150, 152, 155, 166	155	
Lower torso	181, 195, 197, 207, 213, 223-225	223	
Upper back	227, 229	229	
Neck	231, 232, 242, 246	242	
Pectorals	249, 250, 252, 255, 256	252	
Shoulders	258, 269, 271, 276, 280	269	
Arms and wrists	295, 298, 304, 306, 308, 310	298	

IN-LINE SKATING

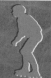

BODY PART	STRETCH NUMBER	BEST	
Feet and ankles	1, 7, 10	10	
Lower legs	13, 19, 21, 28, 30, 41, 42	19	
Hamstrings	50, 53, 55, 63, 65, 70	50	
Adductors	83, 85, 87, 94, 105, 107, 111, 117	94	
Quadriceps	119-121, 131, 132, 134	134	
Hips and gluteals	137, 138, 146, 147, 152, 155, 160, 161	161	
Lower torso	181, 182, 197, 210, 212, 223	182	
Upper back	227-229	229	
Neck	231, 232, 235, 242, 243, 246	243	
Pectorals	248-250, 252	250	
Shoulders	258, 268, 269, 271, 278, 280, 285	269	
Arms and wrists	295, 297-300, 304, 305, 308-311	298	

JOGGING

BODY PART	STRETCH NUMBER	BEST	
Feet and ankles	2, 3, 6, 8, 10	3	
Lower legs	16, 18, 23, 24, 26, 31, 39, 48	23	
Hamstrings	50, 53-55, 65, 70	50	
Adductors	84, 87, 88, 93-96, 117	88	
Quadriceps	119-122, 131, 132, 134	122	
Hips and gluteals	138, 143, 146, 161, 165, 166, 168	161	
Lower torso	181, 182, 197, 204, 209, 213	197	
Upper back	227, 229	227	
Neck	231, 232, 243, 246	231	
Pectorals	248, 250-253	252	
Shoulders	258, 269, 279, 285	269	
Arms and wrists	295, 297, 298, 304, 308, 310	295	

LACROSSE

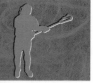

BODY PART	STRETCH NUMBER	BEST	
Feet and ankles	3, 6-8, 10	3	
Lower legs	11, 19, 20, 23, 28, 31, 41	19	
Hamstrings	50, 53, 55, 63, 65, 70	50	
Adductors	82-84, 87, 88, 94, 104, 105, 111, 117	88	
Quadriceps	121-124, 127, 131, 134	121	
Hips and gluteals	137, 138, 146, 147, 155-157, 174	157	
Lower torso	181, 182, 197, 209, 210, 222, 223	223	
Upper back	226, 227, 229	229	
Neck	231, 232, 242, 243, 246	243	
Pectorals	250, 252, 255	252	
Shoulders	258, 269, 271, 272, 274, 275, 279, 280	269	
Arms and wrists	294, 295, 298, 302, 304, 306, 308	298	

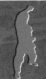

MARTIAL ARTS
beginning

BODY PART	STRETCH NUMBER	BEST	
Feet and ankles	3-5, 7, 9, 10	7	
Lower legs	11, 13, 20, 21, 23, 41	21	
Hamstrings	50-53, 55, 58, 63, 65, 70	58	
Adductors	83, 87, 88, 93-95, 105, 114, 116	93	
Quadriceps	119, 120, 127, 131, 133-135	127	
Hips and gluteals	147, 152, 155-157, 161, 165, 177	161	
Lower torso	181, 182, 184, 185, 197, 199, 207, 210, 221	182	
Upper back	226-228	226	
Neck	231, 232, 235, 243, 246, 247	235	
Pectorals	248-250, 252, 254	252	
Shoulders	258, 269, 271, 276, 282, 285, 290	258	
Arms and wrists	294, 295, 298-300, 304, 305, 308, 311	299	

MARTIAL ARTS
advanced

BODY PART	STRETCH NUMBER	BEST
Feet and ankles	3-5, 8-10	4
Lower legs	21, 23, 24, 29, 43	21
Hamstrings	50, 55, 56, 58-62, 66-68	60
Adductors	88, 90-93, 95, 99, 103, 112-116	103
Quadriceps	126, 127, 130, 131, 133-135	130
Hips and gluteals	148, 158, 160, 162, 173-177	160
Lower torso	182, 184-189, 203, 210, 215, 222	185
Upper back	226, 227, 229	226
Neck	235-238, 243, 246, 247	238
Pectorals	250, 252, 255	250
Shoulders	259, 264, 269, 282, 288-291	269
Arms and wrists	294, 298-302, 308-311	300

RACE WALKING

BODY PART	STRETCH NUMBER	BEST	
Feet and ankles	1-8	7	
Lower legs	11, 13, 15, 21-23, 28, 33, 43-45, 47	22	
Hamstrings	50, 53-55, 63, 69, 80	50	
Adductors	83-85, 87, 88, 96, 105, 111	87	
Quadriceps	119-121, 126, 127, 131, 134	122	
Hips and gluteals	137, 139, 143, 146, 152, 160-162, 170, 174	162	
Lower torso	181-183, 197, 204, 209, 210, 213, 218	182	
Upper back	226, 227, 229, 230	227	
Neck	231, 232, 234, 243, 246	232	
Pectorals	248-250, 252, 254, 255	250	
Shoulders	258, 269, 276, 278-280, 285	280	
Arms and wrists	295, 298-300, 304, 305, 308	299	

ROWING, KAYAKING, AND CANOEING

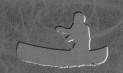

BODY PART	STRETCH NUMBER	BEST	
Feet and ankles	1, 4, 7, 8, 10	7	
Lower legs	13, 19, 21, 28, 29, 31, 32, 40, 47	32	
Hamstrings	50, 51, 53, 63, 65, 69, 80, 81	50	
Adductors	83, 85, 88, 91, 92, 96, 104, 105, 118	91	
Quadriceps	121, 125, 127, 133, 134	125	
Hips and gluteals	137, 143, 152, 154, 159, 161, 173, 174	159	
Lower torso	182, 195, 199, 204, 209, 210, 224, 225	182	
Upper back	227, 229	229	
Neck	231, 232, 239, 240, 243, 244, 246	231	
Pectorals	249, 251-253, 255, 256	252	
Shoulders	260, 261, 264, 266, 269, 280, 282, 290, 291, 293	280	
Arms and wrists	295-304, 306, 308, 310	299	

SAILING AND WINDSURFING

BODY PART	STRETCH NUMBER	BEST	
Feet and ankles	2, 3, 4, 7, 10	4	
Lower legs	13, 20, 21, 23, 24, 28, 29, 41, 47	28	
Hamstrings	50, 53, 55, 63, 69, 70, 79, 80, 81	50	
Adductors	83, 85-87, 91, 96, 104, 105, 109, 117	87	
Quadriceps	119-121, 131, 134	121	
Hips and gluteals	137, 138, 143, 151, 154, 155, 166, 170	155	
Lower torso	181, 182, 195, 211-213, 224, 225	213	
Upper back	227-229	229	
Neck	231, 232, 234, 239, 240, 243, 244, 246	243	
Pectorals	248-250, 252, 255	249	
Shoulders	261, 264, 269, 276, 278, 280, 290	269	
Arms and wrists	295-304, 306, 308, 310	295	

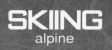

BODY PART	STRETCH NUMBER	BEST	
Feet and ankles	7, 9, 10	9	
Lower legs	13, 17, 20, 21, 24, 27-31, 39, 42	30	
Hamstrings	50-53, 63, 65, 69, 70, 79-81	53	
Adductors	85-88, 91, 93, 94, 105, 117	94	
Quadriceps	119-124, 133-135	123	
Hips and gluteals	138, 147, 151, 152, 155, 161, 162, 166	162	
Lower torso	181, 182, 184, 195, 204, 208, 224, 225	204	
Upper back	226-229	229	
Neck	231, 232, 235, 237, 243, 246	235	
Pectorals	249, 250, 252, 255	250	
Shoulders	261, 268, 269, 278-280, 285, 290	269	
Arms and wrists	295, 297-302, 304, 306, 308, 309	299	

SOCCER
international football

BODY PART	STRETCH NUMBER	BEST	
Feet and ankles	2-4, 6, 8	4	
Lower legs	11, 16, 19, 21, 23, 31, 41	21	
Hamstrings	50, 53-55, 63, 65, 70	55	
Adductors	83, 84, 87, 91, 93-95, 105, 111, 117, 118	94	
Quadriceps	119-121, 124, 127, 131, 134	124	
Hips and gluteals	136, 137, 143, 146, 148, 150, 161, 162, 177	161	
Lower torso	182, 199, 201, 209, 210	201	
Upper back	227, 229, 230	227	
Neck	231, 232, 243, 246	231	
Pectorals	249, 250, 252, 254, 255	252	
Shoulders	259, 272, 285, 290, 293	285	
Arms and wrists	295, 298-300, 304, 308, 309	300	

SQUASH

BODY PART	STRETCH NUMBER	BEST	
Feet and ankles	1, 3, 4, 6-8, 10	3	
Lower legs	12, 16, 19, 21, 24, 47	24	
Hamstrings	50, 53, 55, 63, 65, 70	55	
Adductors	82-84, 88, 94, 95, 105, 109, 117	83	
Quadriceps	119-121, 124, 132, 134	121	
Hips and gluteals	137, 138, 146, 151, 155, 165, 166, 172	165	
Lower torso	181, 182, 196, 197, 204, 207, 209, 222, 223	197	
Upper back	226, 227, 229, 230	229	
Neck	231, 232, 242, 243, 246	243	
Pectorals	249, 250, 252, 255	252	
Shoulders	259, 264, 269, 272, 274, 278, 280, 285	280	
Arms and wrists	294, 295, 298-302, 304, 306, 308, 309	300	

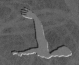

SWIMMING

BODY PART	STRETCH NUMBER	BEST
Feet and ankles	4-10	9
Lower legs	21, 23, 25, 28-31, 47	21
Hamstrings	50, 51, 53, 56, 63, 65	51
Adductors	84-88, 93, 104-107, 111, 114	88
Quadriceps	121, 131, 133-135	134
Hips and gluteals	137, 160-163, 174, 177	160
Lower torso	178, 180-182, 188, 194, 215	181
Upper back	226-230	226
Neck	231, 232, 235, 237, 243, 246	237
Pectorals	250, 255, 256	250
Shoulders	259, 267, 269, 272, 280, 284, 286, 290	284
Arms and wrists	295, 298-301, 304, 308	300

TABLE TENNIS

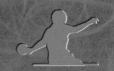

BODY PART	STRETCH NUMBER	BEST	
Feet and ankles	1-5, 7, 8, 10	3	
Lower legs	19, 21, 23, 28, 32, 42, 48	21	
Hamstrings	50, 53, 55, 56, 63, 65, 70	50	
Adductors	87, 88, 90, 91, 93-95, 105, 111, 117	95	
Quadriceps	121, 126, 127, 131, 134	126	
Hips and gluteals	137, 138, 148, 152, 155, 157, 162, 172	157	
Lower torso	181, 182, 194, 197, 204, 212, 215, 221	182	
Upper back	227, 229, 230	227	
Neck	231, 232, 242, 243, 246	242	
Pectorals	250-254	250	
Shoulders	258, 259, 267, 269, 272, 277, 279, 280, 285	267	
Arms and wrists	295, 298, 302, 304, 306, 308, 311	295	

TENNIS, RACQUETBALL, AND HANDBALL

BODY PART	STRETCH NUMBER	BEST	
Feet and ankles	2-5, 7	4	
Lower legs	11, 12, 17, 21, 23, 24, 29, 42	23	
Hamstrings	50, 53-55, 63, 65, 70	53	
Adductors	83, 86, 87, 91, 94, 95, 111, 117	95	
Quadriceps	119-121, 127, 134	121	
Hips and gluteals	138, 148, 150, 152, 155, 166, 172	152	
Lower torso	181-183, 195, 197, 210, 215, 221, 222	182	
Upper back	227, 229, 230	227	
Neck	231, 232, 243, 246	243	
Pectorals	249, 250, 252, 255	249	
Shoulders	259, 267, 269, 271, 272, 278, 280, 286	280	
Arms and wrists	295, 298-302, 304, 306, 308-311	299	

TRACK AND FIELD
high jump and pole vault

BODY PART	STRETCH NUMBER	BEST	
Feet and ankles	2-4, 6, 7, 10	4	
Lower legs	14, 18, 21-23, 26, 39, 40, 48	21	
Hamstrings	50, 53, 55, 56, 65, 66, 80, 81	53	
Adductors	88, 90, 93-95, 97, 98, 105, 114, 117, 118	93	
Quadriceps	124-126, 131, 134	126	
Hips and gluteals	137-139, 142, 143, 152, 161, 162, 174	138	
Lower torso	180-182, 188, 195, 201-203, 210, 215, 224	182	
Upper back	227, 229, 230	227	
Neck	231, 237, 239, 240, 243, 244, 246	237	
Pectorals	249, 250, 253-256	253	
Shoulders	259, 266, 269, 274, 275, 280, 285, 290-293	285	
Arms and wrists	295, 296, 298-304, 306, 308, 309	299	

TRACK AND FIELD
hurdles, long- and triple-jumps, and sprints

BODY PART	STRETCH NUMBER	BEST	
Feet and ankles	1-8, 10	4	
Lower legs	16-18, 20, 21, 31, 32, 42	21	
Hamstrings	50, 51, 53, 55, 56, 80, 81	51	
Adductors	83, 88, 93-95, 114, 117, 118	95	
Quadriceps	121, 125, 134	125	
Hips and gluteals	146, 155, 161, 162, 170	161	
Lower torso	182, 184, 197, 204, 213	182	
Upper back	227, 229, 230	227	
Neck	231, 232, 243, 246	231	
Pectorals	250, 252, 253	250	
Shoulders	259, 269, 279, 280, 285	269	
Arms and wrists	295, 299, 304, 308	299	

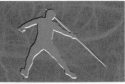

BODY PART	STRETCH NUMBER	BEST	
Feet and ankles	2, 3, 7, 10	3	
Lower legs	13, 21, 23, 31, 43	21	
Hamstrings	50, 53, 55, 80, 81	50	
Adductors	87, 94, 95, 117, 118	94	
Quadriceps	126, 127, 134	126	
Hips and gluteals	137, 138, 146, 169, 170	170	
Lower torso	182, 184, 188, 215, 222, 223, 225	225	
Upper back	227, 229, 230	229	
Neck	232, 233, 239-241, 246	240	
Pectorals	250-253, 255	252	
Shoulders	259, 267, 269, 272, 275, 280, 293	272	
Arms and wrists	295, 299, 304, 306, 308	295	

VOLLEYBALL

BODY PART	STRETCH NUMBER	BEST	
Feet and ankles	2, 3, 6, 7	3	
Lower legs	13, 18, 21, 23, 28, 29, 39, 40, 43, 48	29	
Hamstrings	50, 53, 57, 65, 70, 80, 81	50	
Adductors	83, 88, 92, 93, 105, 117	88	
Quadriceps	121, 122, 124, 131	122	
Hips and gluteals	138, 151, 152, 155-157	156	
Lower torso	181, 195, 197, 211-213, 222	195	
Upper back	227, 229, 230	229	
Neck	231, 242, 243, 246	243	
Pectorals	248, 250, 253, 255	253	
Shoulders	258, 259, 269, 271, 274, 276, 280, 285, 293	271	
Arms and wrists	295, 298-300, 304, 308	300	

WATER SKIING

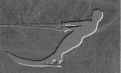

BODY PART	STRETCH NUMBER	BEST	
Feet and ankles	3, 6, 8	8	
Lower legs	22, 24, 31, 44	31	
Hamstrings	51, 55, 56, 69, 80, 81	51	
Adductors	86, 88, 94, 95, 102, 107, 117	94	
Quadriceps	123, 125-127, 134	126	
Hips and gluteals	147, 152, 155, 160-162, 166, 170	160	
Lower torso	194-196, 207, 212, 213, 223	196	
Upper back	226, 227, 229	227	
Neck	232, 235, 237, 242, 243, 246	243	
Pectorals	250, 252, 254	252	
Shoulders	261, 267, 269, 271, 279, 280, 284	280	
Arms and wrists	294, 295, 299, 300, 304, 306, 308	299	

WEIGHT LIFTING

BODY PART	STRETCH NUMBER	BEST	
Feet and ankles	2, 3, 10	3	
Lower legs	13, 17, 23, 27-30, 42	29	
Hamstrings	50, 53, 63	53	
Adductors	83, 88, 91, 95	88	
Quadriceps	123, 125, 131, 134	125	
Hips and gluteals	138, 148, 152, 153, 155, 157, 172	155	
Lower torso	195, 197, 214, 215, 223	214	
Upper back	226, 227	227	
Neck	231, 232, 243, 246	243	
Pectorals	248, 250, 252	250	
Shoulders	261, 267-269, 271, 276, 280, 284	267	
Arms and wrists	294, 295, 298-300, 306, 308, 310	299	

WEIGHT LIFTING
very light weights

BODY PART	STRETCH NUMBER	BEST	
Feet and ankles	3	3	
Lower legs	39, 40	39	
Hamstrings	80, 81	81	
Adductors	117, 118	117	
Quadriceps	131	131	
Hips and gluteals	142, 143	142	
Lower torso	223-225	224	
Upper back	230	230	
Neck	239, 240, 244	240	
Pectorals	256	256	
Shoulders	266, 275, 293	266	
Arms and wrists	296, 303	303	

WRESTLING

BODY PART	STRETCH NUMBER	BEST
Feet and ankles	2, 4, 6, 8	4
Lower legs	13, 21, 23, 26, 43, 44	21
Hamstrings	50, 55, 63, 65, 81	50
Adductors	88, 90, 107, 113, 117, 118	88
Quadriceps	119, 134, 135	135
Hips and gluteals	136-138, 148, 152, 155, 172	155
Lower torso	185, 188, 196, 202, 210, 213, 222, 224, 225	202
Upper back	226, 227	226
Neck	233, 236-238, 243, 246, 247	237
Pectorals	248, 250, 256	250
Shoulders	258, 261, 269, 271, 282, 293	258
Arms and wrists	294, 295, 298-300, 304, 305, 308-311	300

ILLUSTRATED INSTRUCTIONS FOR 311 STRETCHES

The 311 illustrated stretches that follow are arranged by the muscle group or joints to be stretched. As in part III, I have focused on 12 major categories of muscles and joints, including feet and ankles, lower legs, hamstrings, adductors, quadriceps, hips and gluteals, lower torso, upper back, neck, pectorals, shoulders, and arms and wrists. Within these groups I have organized the stretches by their relative difficulty or risk of injury (least difficult and least risky stretches first). The level of difficulty and risk has been determined by the height of the athlete's center of gravity (COG), the use of a partner, and the use of weights or other mechanical aids during the stretch.

In general, a higher COG during a stretch makes it more difficult to maintain balance or support the body, and there is a greater possibility of injury from a fall. Partner stretching can increase the risk of injury because of the partner's potential to provide excessive resistance, resulting in potential sprains and strains. Using weights or other mechanical aids when stretching can also increase the risk of sprains and strains.

Employ a variety of stretches to facilitate developing optimal flexibility and reduce the risk of injury. Always warm up for at least 10 minutes prior to stretching to increase body temperature. The warm-up should be intense enough to induce sweating but not so intense as to cause fatigue. Follow the warm-up with slow static stretches held for 10 to 30 seconds each. Hold the stretch to the point of tension but not pain. Exhale during the stretch to facilitate relaxation during stretching.

Advanced and conditioned athletes may find dynamic, active, or PNF stretching strategies more effective for their needs. Perform dynamic stretches in series, gradually increasing the size of the movements and number of repetitions (up to 8 to 12). Active stretching may be either free active or resistive (manual or mechanical). With active-assisted stretching, the range of motion is completed by a partner or device (inner tube or towel) when one reaches his or her limit of flexibility. PNF techniques include the contract-relax (CR) and contract-relax-agonist-contract (CRAC) methods. CR requires a 6- to 15-second isometric contraction of the muscle(s) to be stretched in a lengthened position. After a brief relaxation, the muscles are further stretched. CRAC is similar to CR except the relaxation phase is followed by an active contraction of the agonist. This text recommends less than maximal isometric contractions to reduce the risk of injury and soreness (see part I for additional details).

Be aware that several of the following stretches may be dangerous for the average person and for an advanced athlete recovering from an injury. These advanced stretches are incorporated specifically for individuals involved in such disciplines as dance, gymnastics, the martial arts, wrestling, and yoga, and they are marked with a cautionary note. Athletes who lack adequate expertise and knowledge should seek out a certified, experienced instructor or trainer. Furthermore, take special care when performing stretches in which the direction of the force is accentuated by a partner. Always communicate with your partner to let him or her know if he or she is stretching you too much and needs to back down. At no time should you compromise your joints' integrity.

Finally, the instructions for the following stretches are written for one side of the body only. Where appropriate, repeat the stretch on the other side. Also watch for caution symbols (see below) accompanying any of the following stretches for special safety instructions.

Before starting any exercise program, have a thorough medical examination. Be examined at regular intervals throughout the program, or any time irregular conditions such as dizziness, pain in the chest, or other symptoms appear. Here are some additional guidelines to follow before beginning a stretching program:

- Identify specific and realistic flexibility goals.
- Do not stretch for approximately 30 minutes after eating.
- Empty your bladder and bowels before stretching.
- Wear loose and comfortable clothing.
- Remove all jewelry.
- Discard all candy and gum.
- Select a clean and quiet place to stretch.
- Work on a nonskid surface—preferably a firm mat.
- Make sure safety comes first. Everyone must be involved in the prevention of injuries.

STRETCHING GUIDELINES

- Warm up prior to stretching.
- Develop a positive mental attitude.
- Isolate the muscle group to be stretched.
- Move slowly and smoothly into the stretch to avoid initiation of the stretch reflex.
- Use proper mechanics and strive for correct alignment.
- Breathe normally and freely, but accentuate exhalation when moving deeper into a stretch.
- Hold a stretch (usually about 10 to 30 seconds) and relax. Do not strain or passively force a joint beyond its normal range of motion.
- Incorporate a progressive velocity flexibility strategy if using dynamic stretches (static > SSER > SFR > FSER > FFR).
- Concentrate and communicate when stretching with a partner.
- Come out of each stretch as carefully as you went into it.

 Stretches marked with this symbol may be dangerous.

FEET AND ANKLES

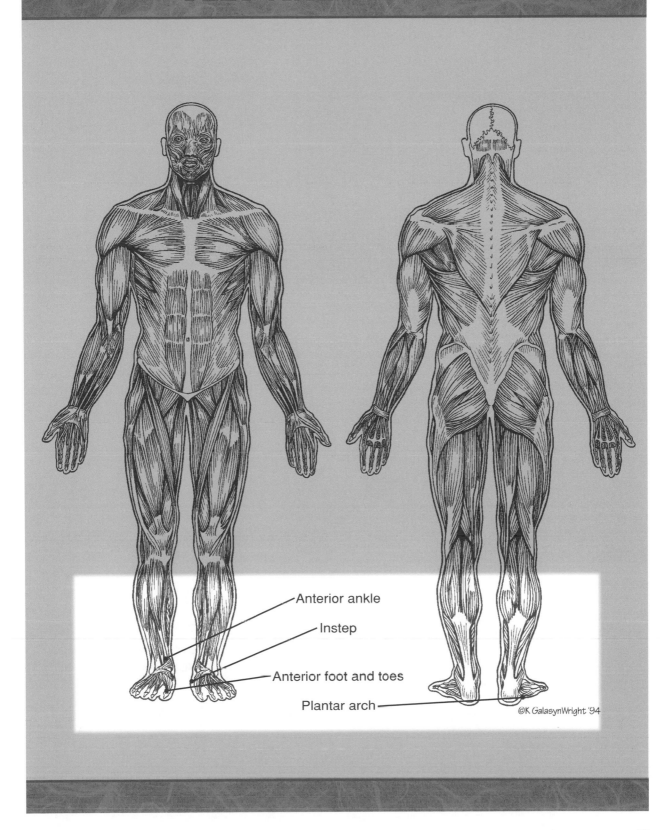

Anterior ankle

Instep

Anterior foot and toes

Plantar arch

©K GalasynWright '94

1

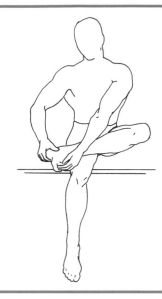

- With one leg crossed over the opposite knee, grasp your ankle with one hand and the underside of your toes and the ball of your foot with your other hand.
- Exhale and pull your toes toward your shins.

2

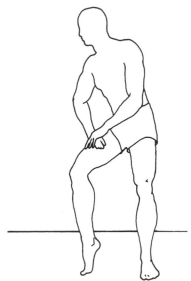

- Stand with one leg slightly in front of the other.
- Exhale, shift your weight onto the ball of your forward foot, and slowly press downward.

3

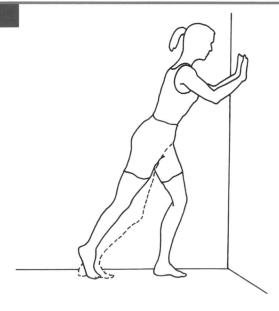

- Standing two to three steps from a wall, bend one leg forward and keep the other leg straight.
- Lean against the wall, keeping your rear foot flat and parallel to your hips.
- Exhale, raise your rear heel off the floor, shift your weight onto the ball of your rear foot, and press downward.

4

- Kneel on all fours with your toes underneath you.
- Exhale and lower your buttocks backward and downward.

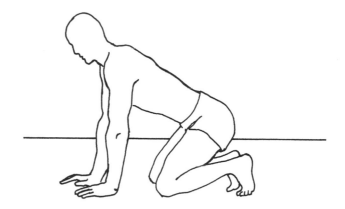

ANTERIOR FOOT AND TOES

5

- Sit with one leg crossed over the opposite knee. Grasp your leg above the ankle with one hand and the top of your foot with your other hand.
- Exhale and pull the bottom of your toes toward the ball of your foot.

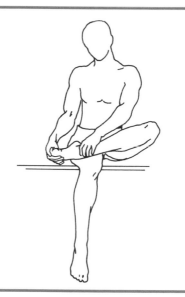

6

- Standing with one leg slightly in front of the other, turn your forward foot under so the top of your toes contacts the floor.
- Exhale, shift your weight forward, and press your toes downward.

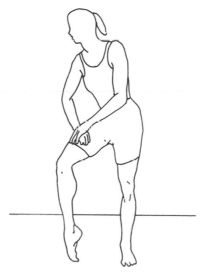

7

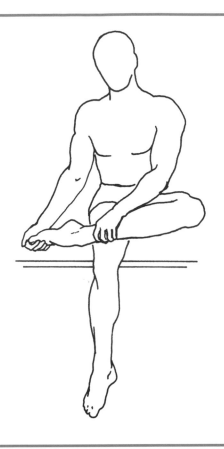

- Sit with one leg crossed over the opposite knee. Grasp your leg above the ankle with one hand and the top of your foot with your other hand.
- Exhale and pull the sole of your foot toward your body.

8

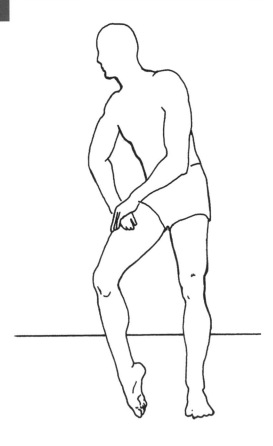

- Standing with one leg in front of the other, turn your forward foot under so the top rests on the floor.
- Exhale, shift your weight forward, and extend the ankle joint.

9

- Kneel with your shins and instep elevated by a cushion or folded mat and your toes pointing backward.
- Exhale and sit on the top of your heels (if you can).

⚠ Be sure your buttocks sit on top of your heels and not between your feet. The latter position is called *W sitting* and is bad for the knees. Do not do this stretch if you have knee problems.

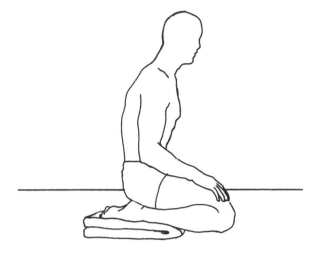

10

- Sit with one leg crossed over the opposite knee. Grasp your leg above the ankle with one hand and the top outside of your foot with the other hand.
- Exhale and slowly invert your ankle (turn your ankle upward).

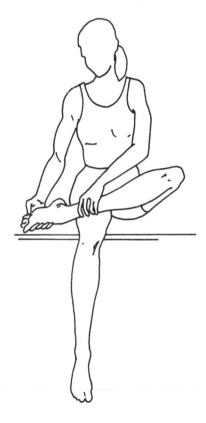

LOWER LEGS

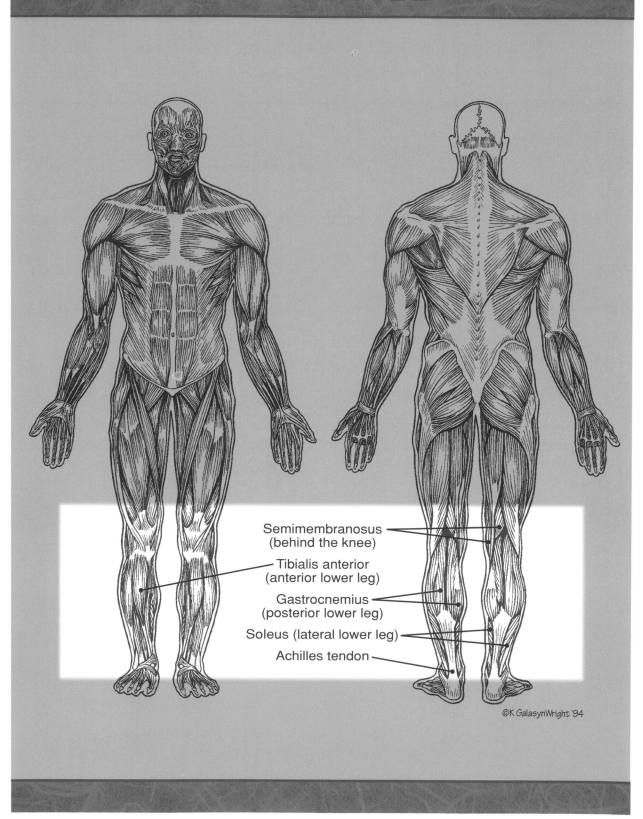

Semimembranosus
(behind the knee)

Tibialis anterior
(anterior lower leg)

Gastrocnemius
(posterior lower leg)

Soleus (lateral lower leg)

Achilles tendon

©K GalasynWright '94

11

- Sit on the floor and flex one knee so that the heel touches the inner side of the opposite thigh.
- Press the outer thigh and calf of the bent leg onto the floor.
- Exhale, keep the extended leg straight, bend at the hips to grasp your foot, and slowly invert your ankle (turn your ankle upward).

NOTE If you are unable to reach your foot, wrap a folded towel around your foot and grasp the ends of it.

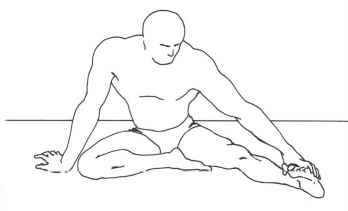

12

- Stand with one or both hands on your hips, using a wall for balance, if necessary.
- Turn one foot under so that the top outside portion rests on the floor.
- Exhale and slowly invert your ankle (turn your ankle upward) and press your foot downward.

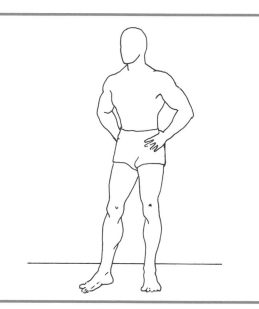

13

- Sit on the floor with both legs spread. Exhale, bend forward at the hips, and grasp both feet.
- Exhale and slowly invert both ankles (turn both ankles upward).

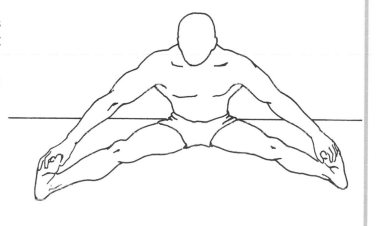

14

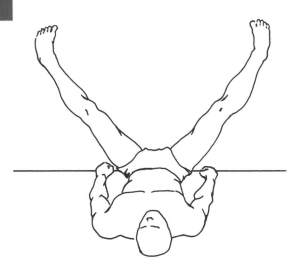

- Lie on your back with your buttocks against a wall and both legs raised and spread.
- Exhale and slowly invert both ankles (turn the outside of both ankles upward).

15

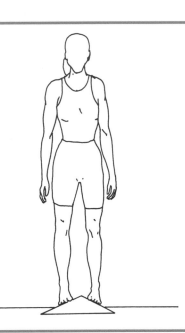

- Stand on an incline board cut at a 45-degree angle.
- Feel the stretch in the anterior and lateral lower leg.

16

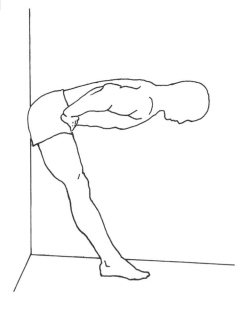

- With your back against a wall and your hands on your hips, slide your feet away from the wall, turn your toes inward, and invert the ankles.
- Exhale and flex forward at the hips; return to the starting position.

⚠️ If you have a "bad back," at the end of the stretch, round your upper torso rather than lifting up with an arched back.

17

- Standing two steps from a pillar, grasp the pillar with both hands, spread your feet (hip-width), and point your toes inward.
- Exhale, flex at the hips, and shift your hips backward, forming a 45-degree angle with your legs.

 Bend your knees when returning to an upright position.

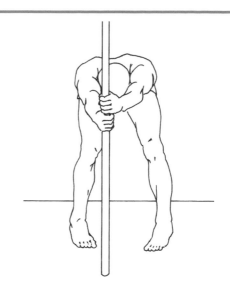

18

- Kneel with your toes pointing backward, exhale, and sit on top of your heels. (If this position is uncomfortable, place a blanket under your shins.)
- Grasp the top portion of your toes and pull them toward your head.

 NOTE Feel the stretch along the shin (tibialis anterior). This stretch can prevent shin-splints.

Be sure your buttocks sit on top of your heels and not between your feet. Do not do this stretch if you have knee problems.

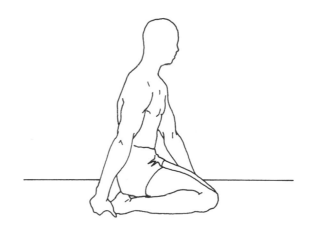

ACHILLES TENDON AND POSTERIOR LOWER LEG

19

- Lying on your back, flex one leg and slide the foot toward your buttocks.
- Raise the opposite leg toward your face, grasp behind the knee, and slowly dorsiflex the foot toward your face.

 NOTE If you have back problems, after the stretch, flex the extended leg and lower it to the floor.

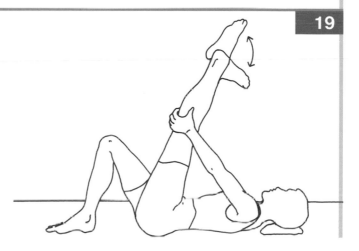

20

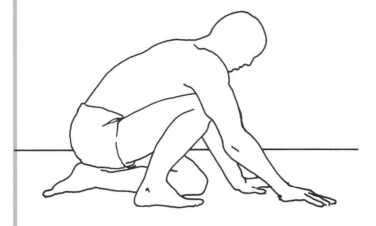

- Kneeling, shift one foot slightly forward and place it flat on the floor.
- Exhale and slowly lean your knee beyond the toes.

21

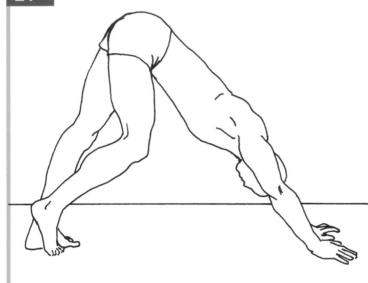

- From a push-up position, move your hands closer to your feet to raise your hips and form a triangle. This position can also be modified by resting your elbows or head on the floor.
- At the highest point of the triangle, slowly press your heels to the floor, or alternate slowly flexing one knee while keeping your opposite leg extended.

22

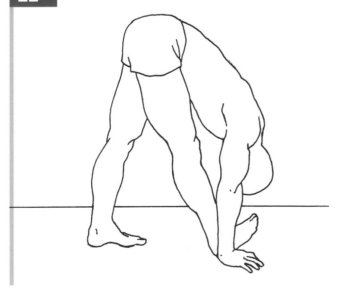

- Stand with your right heel about 12 inches (30 centimeters) in front of the toes of your left foot.
- Flex your right foot toward your shin (dorsiflexion) with the heel in contact with the floor.
- Exhale, lean forward at the hips, and try to touch your right foot with your hands and your leg with your chest while keeping both legs straight.

- Lean against a wall with one leg bent forward and the opposite leg straight.
- Keep your rear heel flat on the floor with the foot pointing straight ahead.
- Exhale, bend your arms and knees, sink your hips, and slowly shift your weight downward onto your rear foot.

 NOTE Keep your rear foot pointed straight ahead with your heel flat on the floor.

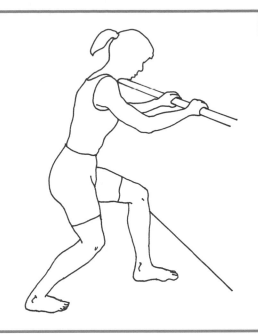

 NOTE Remember in stretches 24 and 25 to start the stretch keeping your head, neck, spine, pelvis, rear leg, and ankle in a straight line.

- Lean forward against a wall with one leg bent forward and the opposite leg straight.
- Keep your rear foot flat on the floor and both feet pointing straight forward. Bend your arms, lean toward the wall, and shift your weight forward.
- Exhale and flex your forward knee toward the wall.

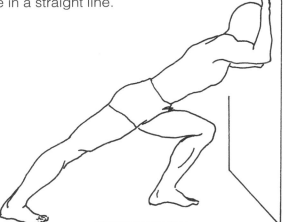

- Lean forward against a wall with one leg bent and the other leg straight with the heel raised.
- Exhale, bend your arms, lean toward the wall, and slowly shift your weight forward while attempting to press your rear heel to the floor.

 NOTE This stretch also effectively stretches the tissues behind the knee.

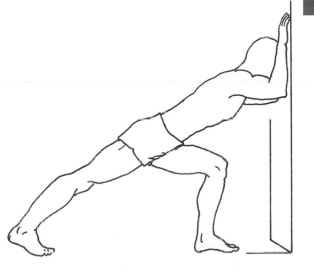

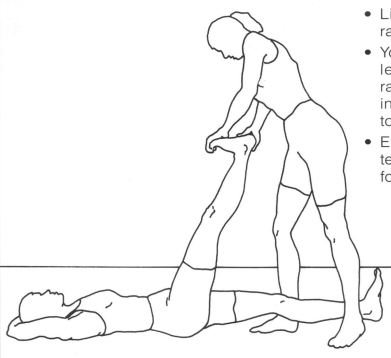

- Lie on your back with one leg raised.
- Your partner straddles your lower leg, grasping the heel of one raised foot with one hand and curling the opposite hand over the toes and ball of the foot.
- Exhale and keep your leg extended as your partner flexes your foot.

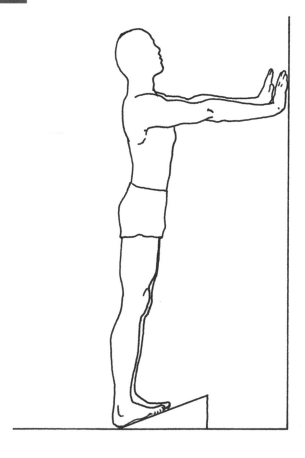

- With the high end of an incline board about an arm's length away from and facing a wall, stand on the board with your hands flat against the wall and lean forward.

NOTE You should feel this stretch in your calves, Achilles tendons, and behind your knees.

- Stand with your hands on your hips or knees.
- Keep your heels on the floor and parallel to one another.
- Exhale, flex your knees, sink your hips, and slowly shift your weight downward while keeping both feet flat on the floor.

NOTE This is an important stretch for those involved in racquet sports.

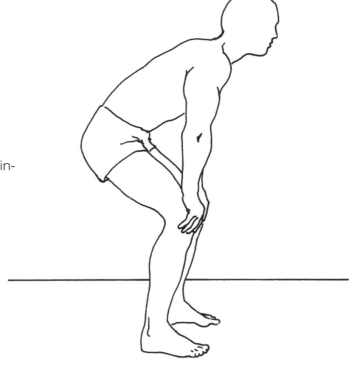

29

- Stand with the balls of your feet balanced on an edge or step.
- Exhale and lower your heels to the floor.

NOTE If necessary, place one hand against a wall for balance and support.

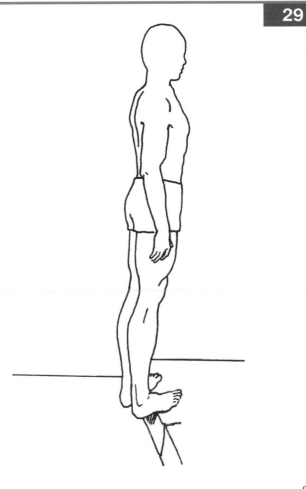

30

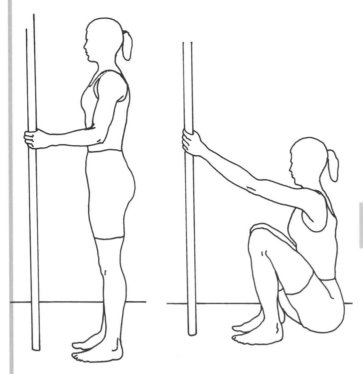

- Holding onto a pole for support, stand with your feet parallel and about 12 inches (30 centimeters) apart.
- Exhale and lean backward, keeping your heels on the floor and your knees behind your toes.
- Squat as low as you can. Exhale while returning to the starting position.

NOTE This stretch may also be felt in tight adductors and quadriceps.

31

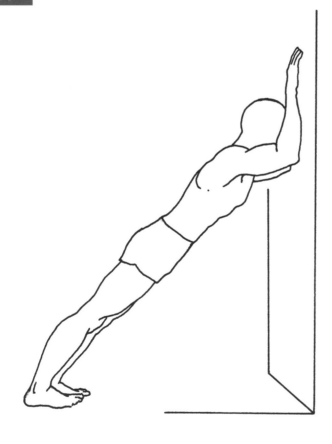

- Lean against a wall, keeping your head, neck, spine, pelvis, legs, and ankles in a straight line.
- Keep your feet flat on the floor and pointing straight ahead.
- Exhale, bend your arms, lean toward the wall, and shift your weight forward.

- Lean against a wall, keeping your head, neck, spine, pelvis, legs, and ankles in a straight line.
- Keep your heels raised and your feet together and pointing straight ahead.
- Exhale, bend your arms, and shift your weight toward the wall while you attempt to press your heels to the floor.

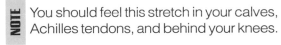

NOTE You should feel this stretch in your calves, Achilles tendons, and behind your knees.

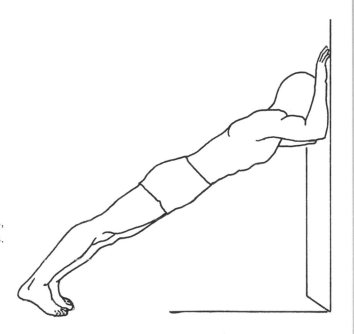

- Standing an arm's length from an open door, grasp the door handles with both hands.
- Balancing on your heels, exhale, keep both legs straight, and shift your hips backward.

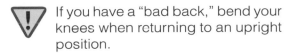

NOTE You should feel this stretch in your calves, Achilles tendons, and behind your knees.

⚠ If you have a "bad back," bend your knees when returning to an upright position.

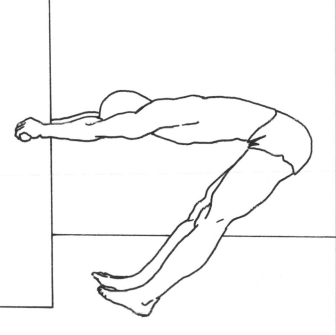

Dance Position Exercises

The following five exercises use the body Positions I through V traditionally used in dance. During these exercises, it is imperative that you avoid initiating the "turnout" from your knees. Instead, concentrate on using your hips and controlling turnout with the interaction between the external and internal rotators of your hip joint. Also focus on equally distributing your weight and keeping your heels flat on the floor. Failure to use proper technique can result in injury to your knees, legs, or feet! You may want to hold onto a barre or chair back for support and balance.

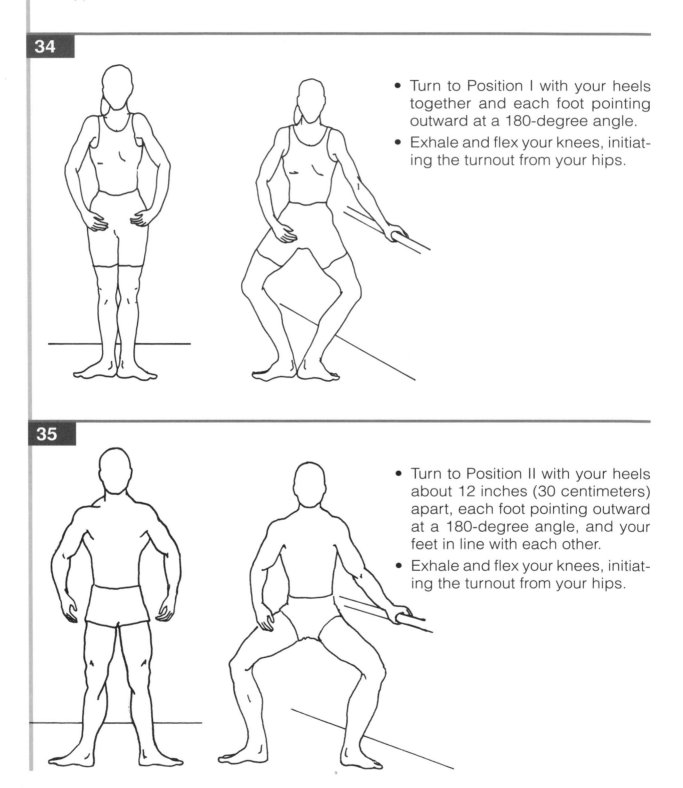

34

- Turn to Position I with your heels together and each foot pointing outward at a 180-degree angle.
- Exhale and flex your knees, initiating the turnout from your hips.

35

- Turn to Position II with your heels about 12 inches (30 centimeters) apart, each foot pointing outward at a 180-degree angle, and your feet in line with each other.
- Exhale and flex your knees, initiating the turnout from your hips.

36

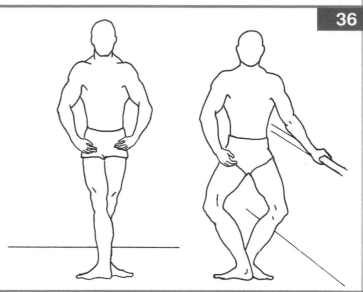

- Turn to Position III so your feet are in line and pressed together, the heel of one foot at the arch or instep of the other foot and the toes pointing in opposite directions.
- Exhale and flex your knees, initiating the turnout from your hips.

37

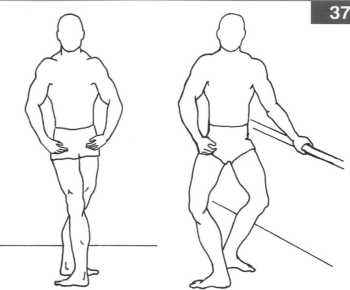

- Turn to Position IV with your feet pointed in opposite directions, one foot approximately 12 inches (30 centimeters) in front of the other and the heel of your forward foot in line with the toes of your back foot.
- Exhale and flex your knees, initiating the turnout from your hips.

38

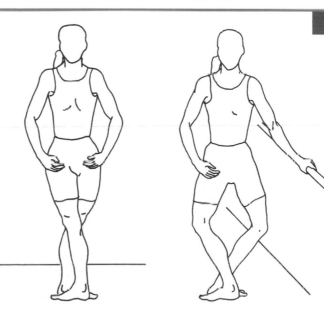

- Turn to Position V with your feet pointed in opposite directions, the heel of your front foot flat against the toe of your other foot and the heel of your rear foot against the toe of your front foot.
- Exhale and flex your knees, initiating the turnout from your hips.

39

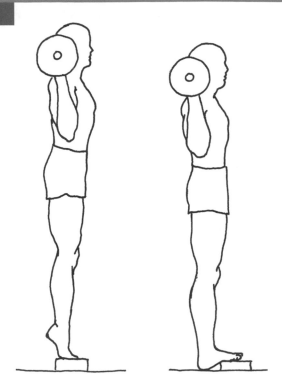

- Stand with your toes and the balls of your feet on a thick board. Rest a lightweight barbell on your shoulders.
- Exhale while rising up on your toes as high as possible.
- Inhale and lower your heels until they almost touch the floor; return to the starting position.

NOTE Use a light weight that you can handle easily.

40

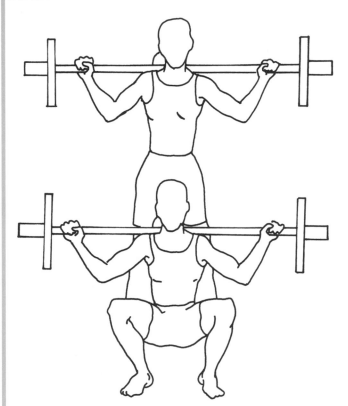

- Stand with your feet about shoulder-width apart and rest a lightweight barbell on your shoulders.
- Inhale and lower your buttocks toward the floor while keeping your heels flat on the floor.
- Hold the stretch at the bottom before exhaling and returning to the starting position.

NOTE Always use a light weight that you can handle easily. A lifting belt can also provide extra support.

⚠ This exercise is essential for weight lifters. Athletes simply seeking to increase strength can protect their knees by lowering the buttocks. This exercise may be too advanced or dangerous for even some elite athletes.

As a general rule, avoid the following stretches if you have hyperextended knees.

41

- Sit on the floor with knees flexed, grasp your toes and the ball of one foot, and extend this leg.
- Exhale; keeping your leg straight, pull your foot toward your trunk and bend at the hip so that your upper torso leans toward the extended thigh.

NOTE Contracting and then relaxing the quadriceps of the extended leg tends to alleviate some tension and discomfort behind the knee. This action will also allow you to lean your upper torso closer to your thigh.

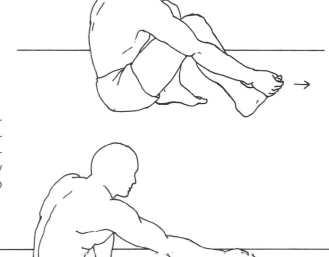

42

- Sitting on the floor with your legs spread, flex one leg inward until its heel touches the groin of the extended leg.
- Exhale, lean forward, and grasp the foot of your extended leg. Keep your leg straight while pulling your foot toward your torso.

NOTE Try contracting and then relaxing the quadriceps on this stretch to alleviate some tension behind the knee.

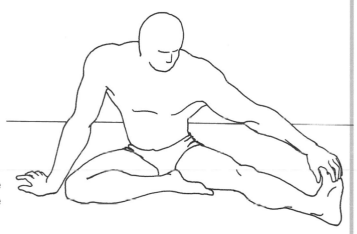

43

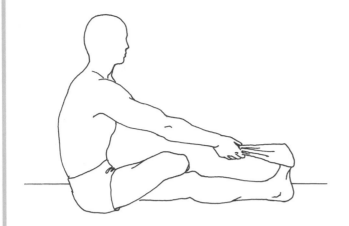

- Sitting on the floor, cross one leg and rest the heel on the opposite knee.
- Hold both ends of a folded towel wrapped around the ball of your extended foot.
- Exhale, keep your extended leg straight, and pull the towel to pull your foot toward your trunk.

NOTE Athletes with adequate flexibility will not need a towel.

44

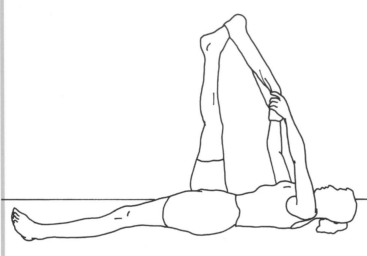

- Lie on your back with your legs extended; grasp both ends of a folded towel.
- Flex one leg over your chest and loop the towel around the ball of your foot.
- Exhale, straighten your knee, and bring your toes toward you as far as possible.
- Keeping your hips squared, legs, back, and head flat on the floor, pull on the towel.

45

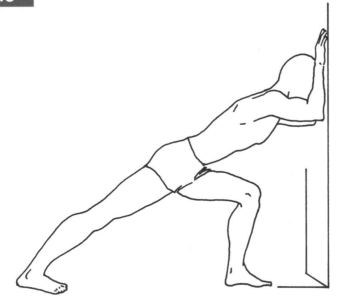

- Standing an arm's length from a wall, bend one leg forward and lean against the wall without losing the straight line of your head, neck, spine, pelvis, rear leg, and ankle.
- Keep your rear foot down and parallel to your hips, bend your arms, and shift your weight toward the wall.
- Exhale and contract the quadriceps of your rear leg without jamming or locking the knee.

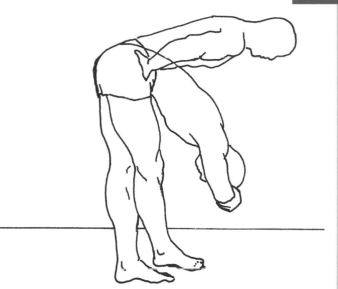

46

- Stand with your hands on your hips and cross one leg over the other.
- Exhale; keeping one leg straight, extend your upper back. Bend at the hips and lower your trunk onto your thigh.

NOTE Bend your knees or round your upper torso rather than lifting with an arched back when returning to an upright position.

NOTE To intensify the stretch, place your arms behind your head, grasping your elbows.

47

- Sitting on the floor with both legs straight, lean forward and grasp your feet with your hands or with a folded towel.
- Slowly pull your feet back toward your trunk.

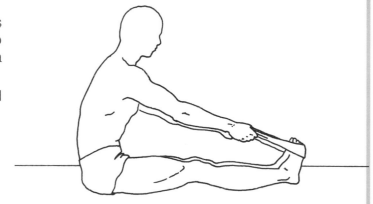

- Standing an arm's length from a wall with your feet shoulder-width apart and toed in, lean against the wall without losing the straight line of your head, neck, spine, pelvis, rear leg, and ankle.
- Keep both heels down and toed in. Bend your arms and lean toward the wall.
- Exhale and contract the quadriceps without jamming or locking the knees.

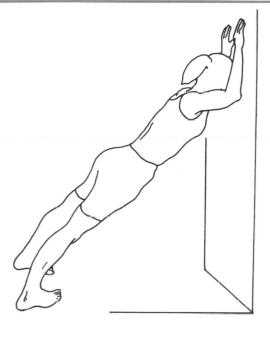

49

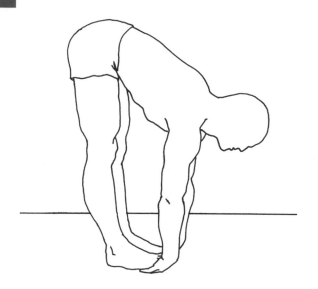

- Standing with both legs straight, exhale and extend your upper back.
- Bend forward at the hips and grasp your toes with your hands. Pull up on your toes.

NOTE Remember to either bend your knees or round your upper torso rather than lifting with an arched back when returning to an upright position. Also, try contracting and then relaxing your quadriceps to alleviate tension behind your knees.

HAMSTRINGS

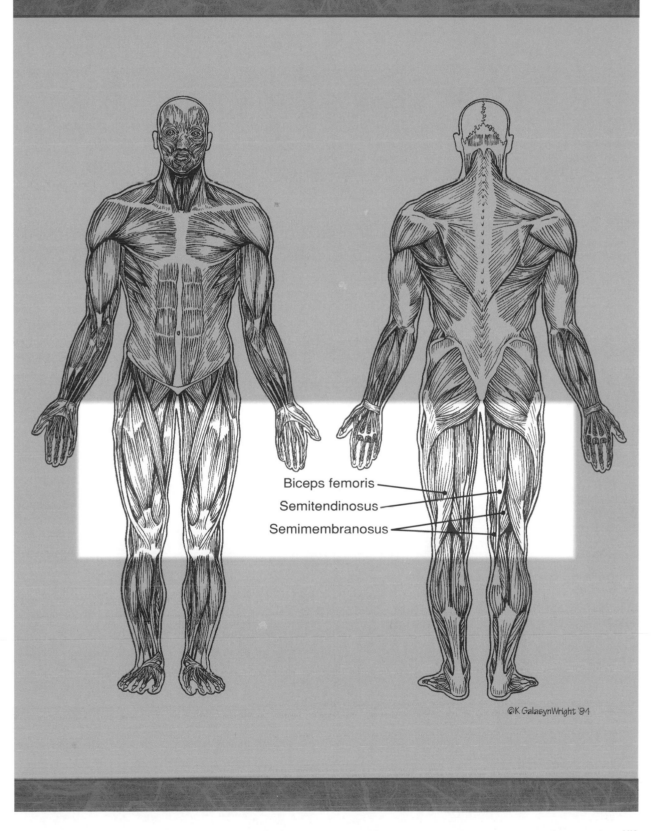

Biceps femoris
Semitendinosus
Semimembranosus

©K. GalasynWright '94

50

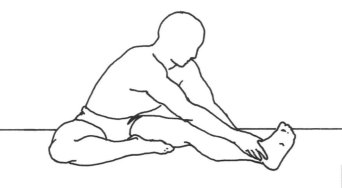

- Sit on the floor with one leg straight and the other bent at the knee with the heel touching the inside of the opposite thigh.
- Lower the outside of the thigh and calf of the bent leg onto the floor.
- Exhale, keep the extended leg straight, and lower your upper torso onto your thigh.

 NOTE Try contracting your quadriceps to alleviate tension in your hamstrings.

51

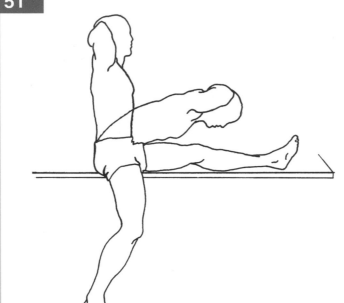

- Sit on a bench with one leg extended and your opposite foot on the floor. Place your hands behind your head.
- Exhale, extend your upper back, flex at the hips, and lower your torso onto your thigh while keeping your elbows raised and your leg straight.

 NOTE Try contracting your quadriceps to alleviate tension in your hamstrings.

52

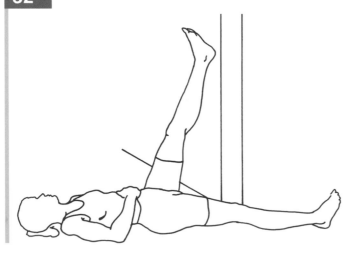

- Lie on your back in a doorway and position your hips slightly in front of the door frame.
- Raise one leg and rest it against the door frame while keeping that knee extended and your bottom leg on the floor. Increase the stretch by sliding your hips closer to the door frame or lifting the leg away from the door frame.

 NOTE Try contracting your quadriceps to alleviate tension in your hamstrings.

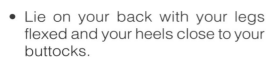

53

- Lie on your back with your legs flexed and your heels close to your buttocks.
- Inhale and extend one leg upward.
- Exhale and slowly pull the raised leg toward your face, keeping the leg straight.

NOTE Try contracting your quadriceps to alleviate tension in your hamstrings. Also, if you have a bad back, flex the extended leg and slowly lower it to the floor.

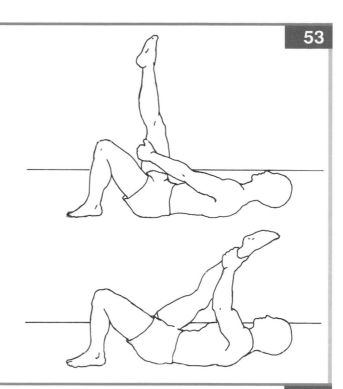

54

- Lying on your back, wrap a folded towel around the instep of one foot, inhale, and extend the leg upward.
- Exhale and pull the raised leg toward your face, keeping the leg straight.

NOTE Try contracting your quadriceps to alleviate tension in your hamstrings. Also, if you have a bad back, flex the extended leg and slowly lower it to the floor.

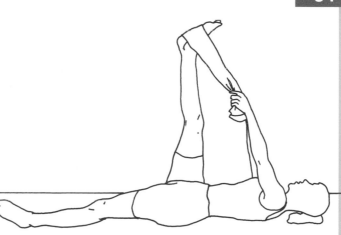

55

- Sit on the floor with your hands behind your hips for support and your legs extended.
- Flex one knee and grasp the instep of your foot with one hand.
- Exhale and extend your leg until it is perpendicular to the floor.

NOTE Try contracting your quadriceps to alleviate tension in your hamstrings.

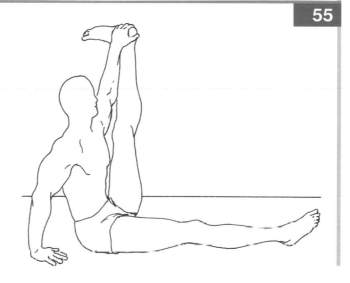

56

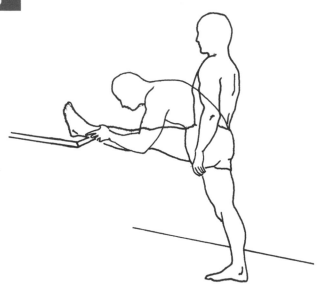

- Standing, slowly raise one leg and rest it on an elevated platform at a comfortable height.
- Exhale; keeping both legs straight and your hips squared, slowly flex forward from the hips, extend your upper back, and lower your trunk onto your raised thigh.

NOTE Try contracting your quadriceps to alleviate tension in your hamstrings.

57

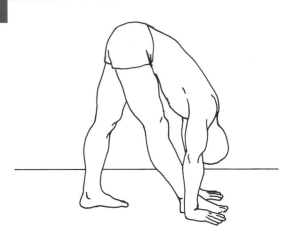

- Stand with your right foot about 12 inches (30 centimeters) in front of the toes of your left foot.
- Exhale, lean forward at the hips, and try to touch the floor or your right foot with your hands while keeping both legs straight.

58

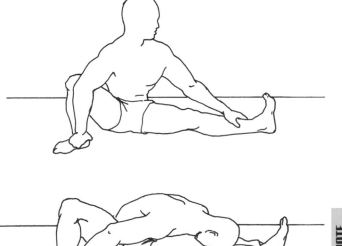

- Assume a squat position with your feet flat on the floor.
- Place your weight on one flexed knee and extend the opposite leg sideways.
- Grasp your right ankle with your right hand and your left ankle with your left hand.
- Exhale and lower your entire upper torso to your extended thigh.

NOTE This exercise is fundamental for martial artists; however, it is not necessary for most other athletes. This exercise also stretches the groin.

59

- Kneeling with both legs together and your hands at your sides, lift one knee and place your foot slightly in front for support.
- Exhale, bend at the hips, lower your upper torso onto the front thigh, and place your hands slightly in front of the front foot.
- Slide your front foot forward and straighten your rear leg as you extend into the split position.

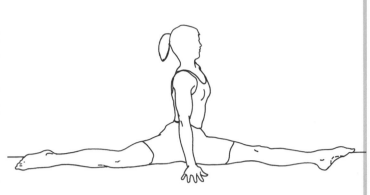

NOTE A split is one of the more advanced stretches for the hamstrings. To perform a technically correct split, both legs must be straight, the hips squared (facing forward, not twisted sideways), and the buttocks flat on the floor. For aesthetic reasons, some advocate a slight turnout of the rear hip. However, due to tight hip flexors or improper training, this turnout can be too extreme.

- Perform a split.
- Exhale and lower your extended upper torso onto the forward thigh.

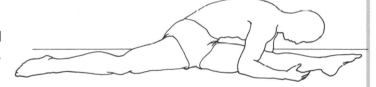

- Kneel with both legs together and your hands on the floor at your sides for balance.
- Lift one knee and place your foot slightly in front of your body on a folded blanket.
- Exhale, slowly slide your front foot forward while resting it on the folded blanket, and straighten your rear leg as you extend into the split position.

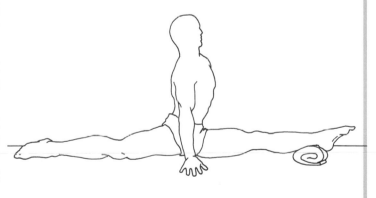

NOTE You should also feel this stretch behind the knee.

⚠️ This exercise is useful for advanced athletes who require exceptional flexibility in their disciplines: pairs figure skating, the martial arts, and rhythmic gymnastics. However, most other athletes should not incorporate this exercise into their stretching program.

62

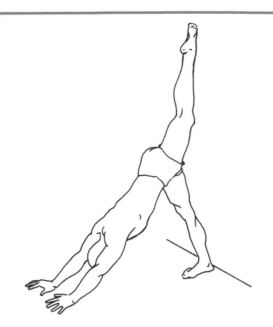

- Stand with your back approximately three feet (one meter) from a wall; bend over and place your hands on the floor for support, and raise one leg against the wall.
- Exhale and slide your leg upward against the wall until you attain the split position with your legs straight and hips squared.

63

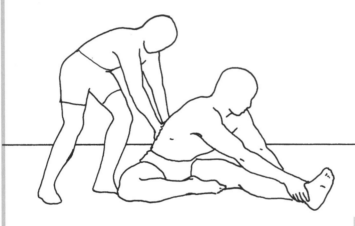

- Sitting on the floor with your legs extended and spread apart, flex one knee until its heel touches the groin of the other leg.
- Your partner stands behind you with one hand in the center of your upper back and the other in the center of your lower back.
- Exhale; keeping your forward leg straight, extend your upper back, and bend forward at the hips as your partner gently pushes your upper torso onto your thigh.

 NOTE Remember to communicate with your stretching partner.

64

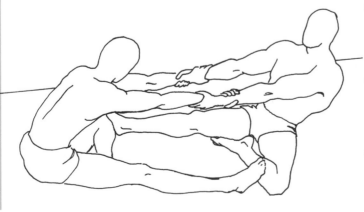

- Sitting on the floor with your legs extended and spread apart, flex one knee until its heel touches the groin of the other leg.
- Your partner assumes the same position while you brace your extended leg against your partner's flexed leg and vice versa; interlock hands.
- Exhale, bend forward at the hips, and lower your trunk onto your extended thigh as your partner leans backward and pulls on your hands.

65

- Lie on your back and raise one leg, keeping your hips square.
- Your partner anchors your leg on the ground and grasps your raised leg.
- Exhale as your partner raises your leg upward.

  Remember to keep both legs straight and your hips squared.

 Your partner should avoid grasping the heel because the leverage may result in straining the knee.

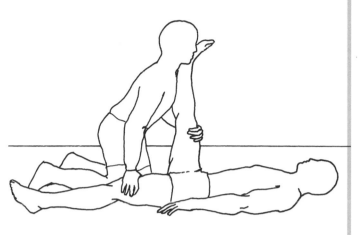

- Stand facing your partner and holding onto a surface for balance.
- Inhale and raise one leg for your partner to grasp with both hands above your ankle.
- Exhale as your partner raises your leg.

NOTE Remember to keep both legs straight and your hips squared. Remember to communicate with your partner.

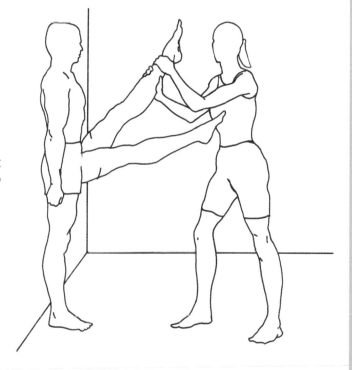

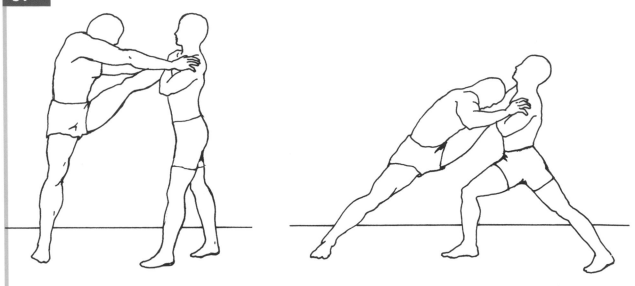

- Stand facing your partner and place one leg on your partner's shoulder.
- Exhale and bend forward to your knee as your partner steps backward.

NOTE This stretch is commonly cited in martial arts texts but is unnecessary for most athletes.

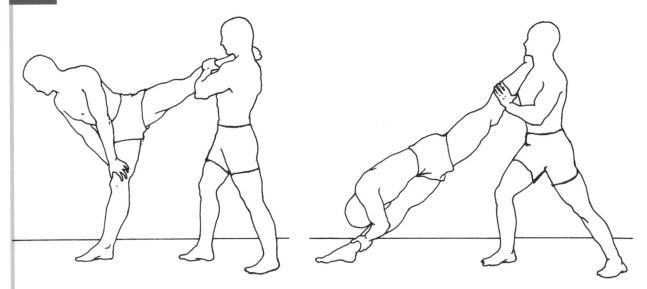

68

- Stand facing your partner and place one leg on your partner's shoulder.
- Turn away from your partner, exhale, and lean toward your ankle as your partner steps backward.

NOTE This stretch is commonly cited in martial arts texts but is unnecessary for most athletes.

69

- Sit on the floor with both legs extended in front of you.
- Exhale; keep your legs straight, extend your upper back, bend forward at the hips, and lower your trunk onto your thighs.

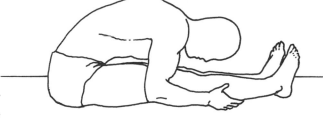

NOTE — You should also feel this stretch in your lower back. Try contracting your quadriceps to alleviate tension in your hamstrings.

70

- Sit on the floor with both legs spread and extended in front of you.
- Exhale; keep your legs straight, extend your upper back, bend forward at the hips, and lower your trunk onto the floor.

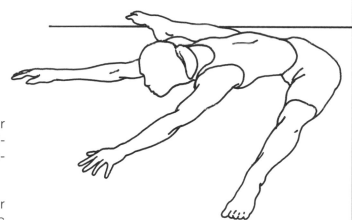

NOTE — You should also feel this stretch in your lower back. Try contracting your quadriceps to alleviate tension in your hamstrings.

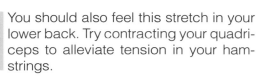 Do not lift your heels off the floor or roll your hips or thighs inward, as this may strain the groin.

71

- Squat with your heels flat, your chest on your thighs, and your hands on the floor for balance.
- Exhale and slowly straighten your legs. Stop when you feel excess tension.
- Flex your knees and return to the starting position.

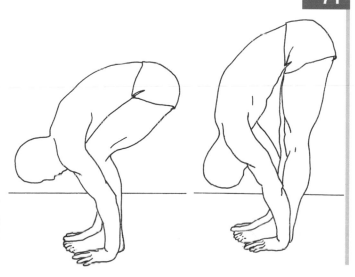

NOTE — You should also feel this stretch in your lower back. You can initiate this stretch with your buttocks resting against a wall for balance.

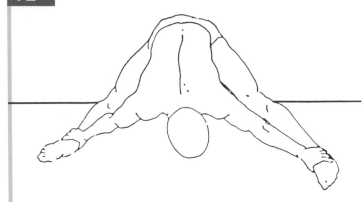

- Stand with your legs spread and flex at the hips, keeping your legs straight. Grasp your ankles or feet.
- Exhale and pull your chest closer to your legs.
- Flex your knees to return to the starting position.

73

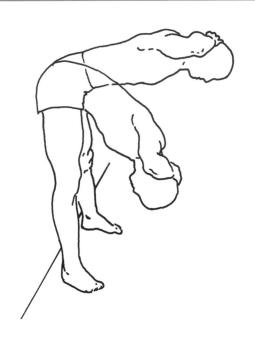

- Stand with your legs spread and the back of your heels approximately 12 inches (30 centimeters) from a wall.
- Interlock your hands behind your head. Keeping your legs straight, extend your upper back, bend forward at the hips, and lower your trunk toward your thighs.
- Exhale and bend your knees or round your upper torso when returning to the upright position.

74

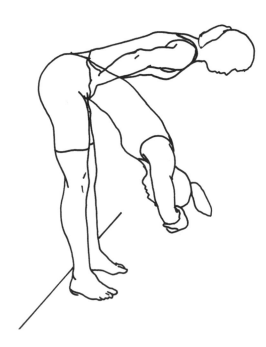

- Stand 12 inches (30 centimeters) from a wall with the back of your heels almost together.
- Interlock your hands on top of your head, bend forward at the hips, and lower your trunk toward your thighs.

- Stand 12 inches (30 centimeters) from a wall with the back of your heels almost together.
- Exhale, bend forward at the hips, lower your trunk toward your thighs, and touch your toes.
- Exhale and bend your knees or round your upper torso when returning to the upright position.

 NOTE Remember to keep your legs straight.

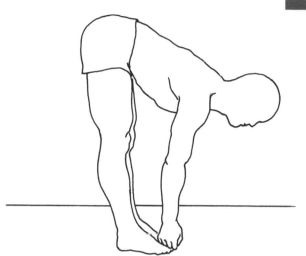

76

- Stand 12 inches (30 centimeters) from a wall with the back of your heels almost together.
- Exhale, bend forward at the hips, lower your trunk toward your thighs, and place your hands flat on the floor.
- Exhale and bend your knees or round your upper torso when returning to the upright position.

 NOTE This stretch is vital for 3- and 10-meter divers.

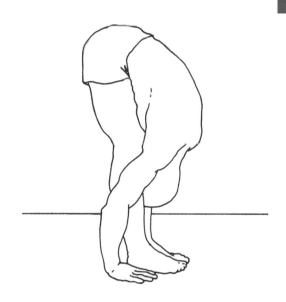

- Stand 12 inches (30 centimeters) from a wall with the back of your heels almost together.
- Exhale, bend forward at the hips, lower your trunk toward your thighs, grasp the backs of your ankles, and slowly compress your upper torso to your thighs.

 NOTE This stretch is vital for 3- and 10-meter divers.

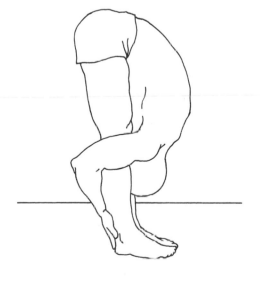

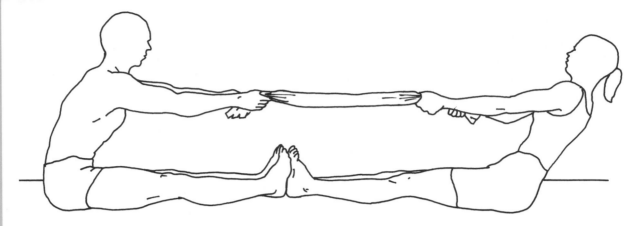

- Sit on the floor with your legs extended. Your partner assumes the same position with feet braced against yours.
- You and your partner each hold one end of a folded towel.
- Exhale; keeping your legs straight, extend your upper back, bend forward at the hips, and lower your trunk onto your thighs as your partner leans backward and pulls on the towel.

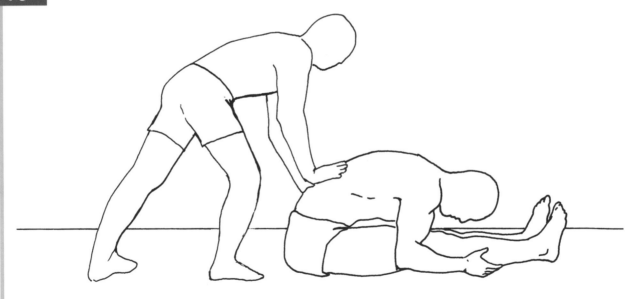

- Sit on the floor with your legs extended while your partner stands behind you with one hand in the center of your upper back and the other in the center of your lower back.
- Exhale; keeping your legs straight, extend your upper torso and bend forward at the hips as your partner pushes your upper torso onto your thighs.

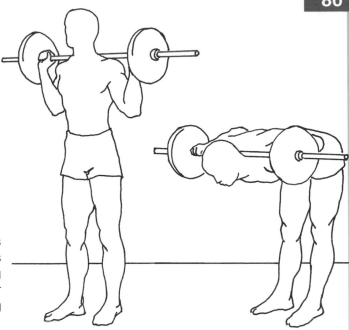

- Stand with your feet shoulder-width apart holding a lightweight barbell on your shoulders.

- Inhale, keep your legs straight, bend at the hips, and lower your upper torso to a horizontal position.

- Hold the stretch momentarily before exhaling and returning to an upright position.

NOTE Some athletes slightly flex their legs when using heavier weights with this exercise. The objective when using heavier weights is to strengthen the lower back. It is a good idea to wear a lifting belt when performing this stretch.

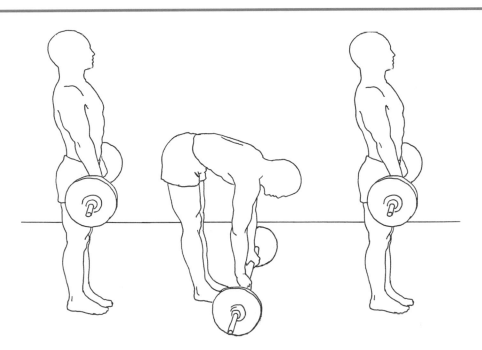

- Stand holding a lightweight barbell with your arms straight in front of you.

- Inhale, keep your legs straight, bend forward at the hips, and lower the barbell to the floor.

- Hold the stretch momentarily, exhale, and slowly return to an upright position.

NOTE This exercise is basic for bodybuilders, power lifters, and weight lifters. As flexibility increases, advanced athletes may want to do these "dead lifts" while standing on the end of a bench or large block.

 Use a lifting belt when doing this lift/stretch.

ADDUCTORS

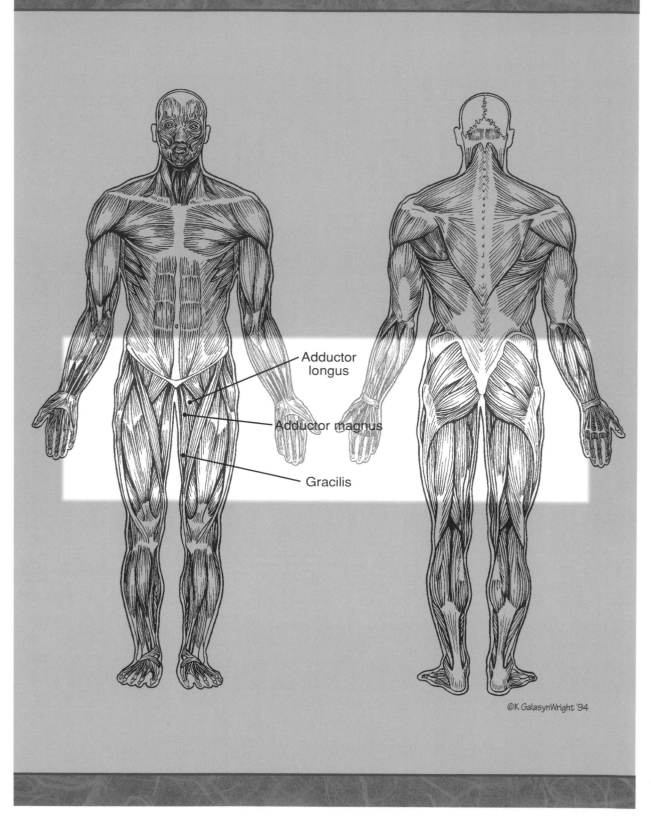

Adductor longus

Adductor magnus

Gracilis

©K GalasynWright '94

- Sit on the floor with your buttocks against a wall, your legs flexed and spread, and your heels touching each other.
- Grasp your feet or ankles and pull them as close to your groin as possible.
- Place your elbows on your inner thighs or knees, exhale, and push your legs to the floor.

NOTE Be sure to keep your back straight when performing this exercise.

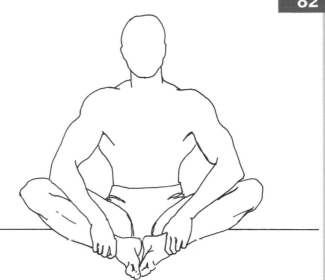

- Sit on the floor with your buttocks against a wall, your legs flexed and spread, and your heels touching each other.
- Grasp your feet or ankles and pull them as close to your groin as possible.
- Exhale and lean forward from the hips. Keep your back straight and attempt to lower your chest to the floor.

NOTE If you have tight adductors, you may find it easier to perform this stretch with your heels extended slightly forward.

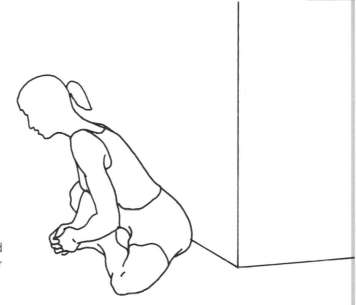

- Lie on your back and flex your knees, bringing the heels and soles of your feet together as you pull them toward your buttocks.
- Exhale and spread your knees as wide as possible, keeping the soles of your feet in contact.

NOTE The stretch will feel more intense if performed on a narrow bench. Focus on moving your upper thighs outward and not your knees. Some athletes will find it useful to wrap a belt around the upper thighs or ankles.

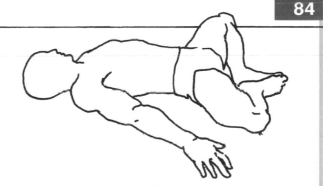

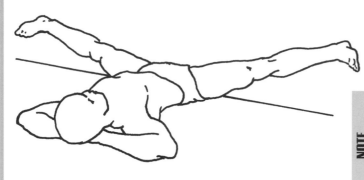

- Lie on your back with your legs raised and together and your buttocks several inches from a wall.
- Exhale and slowly spread your legs as wide as possible.

NOTE This stretch can be intensified by wearing shoes, weighted boots, or placing a small folded towel under your buttocks so your thighs are slightly above their resting position. Placing your hands on the insides of your knees can provide an additional manual stretch.

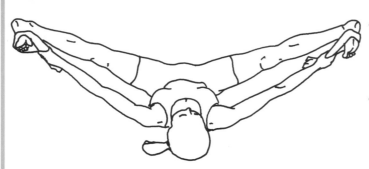

- Lying on your back, loop a pair of straps around both feet at the instep; inhale and extend your legs upward.
- Exhale, spread your legs as wide as possible, and pull on the straps at the end of the movement.

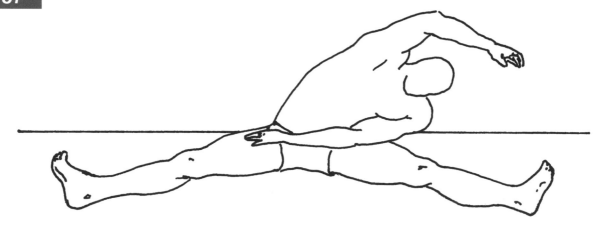

- Sit on the floor with your legs spread as wide as possible.
- Drop one arm and raise your other arm overhead.
- Exhale, rotate your trunk, and bend from the hip, leaning your upper torso onto your leg.

NOTE You may also feel this stretch in the lateral portion of your torso.

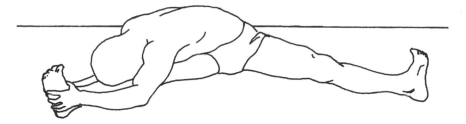

- Sit on the floor and spread your legs as wide as possible.
- Exhale, rotate your trunk, slowly extend your upper torso onto one leg, and grasp your foot.

 NOTE Concentrate on keeping your lower back and legs extended and your heels on the floor.

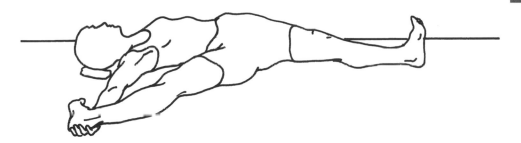

- Lie on your back. Flex one leg, grasp the foot, and extend the leg vertically.
- Exhale and slowly lower your leg to the floor at your side, forming the letter *Y*.

NOTE Be sure to keep your body extended.

- Kneel on all fours with your toes pointing backward. Extend one leg sideways.
- Exhale, bend your arms, lower the hip of the opposite side to the floor, and roll the hip.

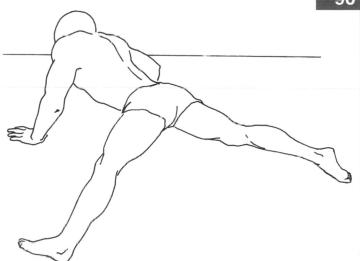

91

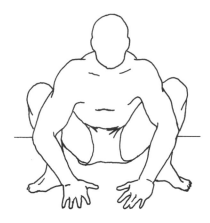

- Squat with your feet flat on the floor about 12 inches (30 centimeters) apart and your toes turned slightly outward.
- Place your elbows on your thighs, exhale, and push your legs outward with your elbows.

NOTE Remember to keep your feet flat on the floor to reduce strain on your knees.

92

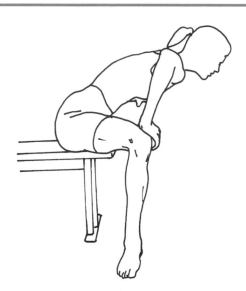

- Sit on the end of a bench with your legs spread slightly wider than hip-width apart, feet flat on the floor, and toes pointing outward at a 180-degree angle (the heels of your feet parallel and facing each other).
- Place your hands on your knees, exhale, flex from the hips, and lower your upper torso toward the floor while keeping your back extended. Use your hands to push your legs outward (abduction).

93

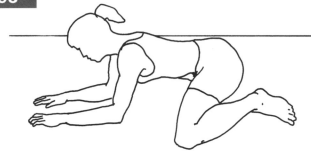
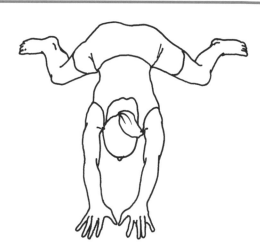

- Kneel with your toes pointing out to the sides; rest your elbows on the floor.
- Exhale, spread your knees, and lower your chest to the floor as you extend your arms parallel and forward.

NOTE This stretch is one of the most intense for the adductors. If you are extremely pliable, you will be able to lower into a straddle split with your knees flexed.

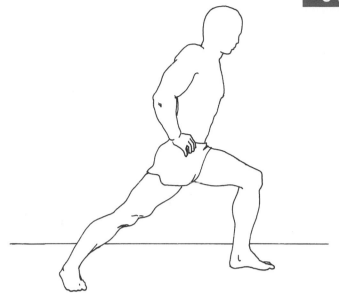

- Stand with your legs spread about two feet (60 centimeters) apart and turn your right foot 90 degrees sideways to the right, keeping your toes and heel in line with your body.
- Place your hands on your hips, exhale, lunge forward with your left leg, and press down on your right hip.

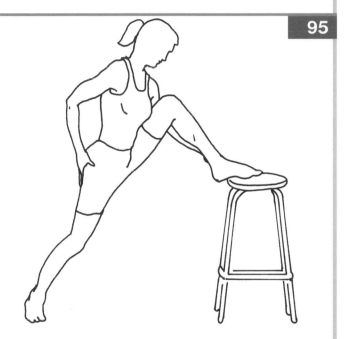

- Stand with one foot on the top surface of a sturdy chair and slide your rear leg backward while holding onto the chair for balance.
- Exhale and lean forward and downward while bending the knee of the leg resting on the chair.

NOTE If a chair is unavailable, use an elevated but sturdy surface.

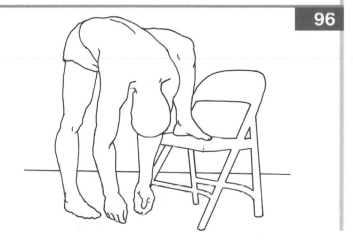

- Stand with one foot resting on the seat of a chair.
- Exhale, bend at the hip, and lower your hands toward the floor.

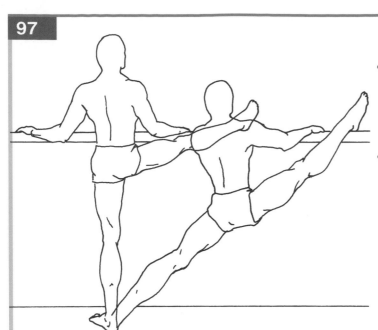

97

- Stand facing a barre or a supporting surface about hip high, inhale, raise one leg to the supporting surface, and place your heel or instep on top.

- Exhale and slide your foot along the surface.

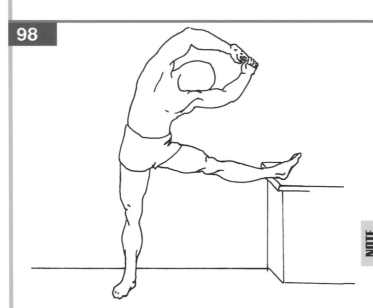

98

- Stand with your feet parallel to a supporting surface of approximately hip height. Place one heel on top of the surface.

- Interlock your hands over your head, exhale, and bend sideways, lowering your upper torso toward your raised thigh.

NOTE Keep your legs straight. You may also feel this stretch in the lateral torso.

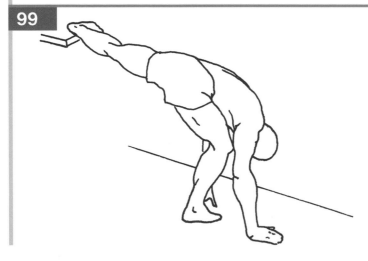

99

- Stand with your feet parallel to a supporting surface of approximately hip height. Keeping both legs straight and your hips squared, place one heel on the supporting surface.

- Turn out the foot of the supporting leg and turn the raised leg medially.

- Exhale, keep the raised leg straight, flex the supporting leg, and lower your chest to your knee.

- Stand with your feet parallel to a supporting surface of approximately hip height. Keeping both legs straight and your hips squared, raise and place your heel on the supporting surface.
- Turn out the foot of the supporting leg and turn the raised leg medially.
- Grasp the raised foot with one hand, bend forward at the hips, and grasp the foot of the supporting leg with your other hand.
- Exhale; keep both legs straight and lower your upper torso as if performing a straddle split.

 NOTE You may also feel this stretch in your hamstrings.

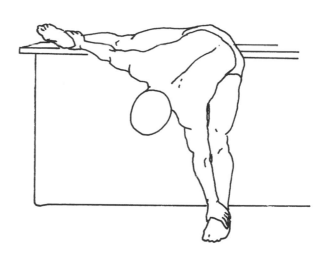

- Standing, draw the toe of one foot to the opposite ankle and slide it up the inside of your leg to your knee.
- Grasp the foot or ankle with your hand, inhale, and raise and straighten your leg sideways.

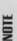 **NOTE** Dancers are capable of performing this skill without using their arms for support. For many, lack of coordination or strength in the hip flexors limits their ability to do this stretch.

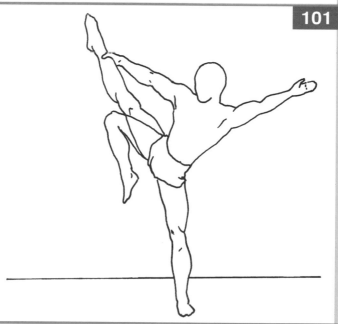

- Sit on the floor with your legs together and extended.
- Exhale and spread your legs to a straddle split position while keeping your upper torso erect.

 NOTE Remember to keep your toes pointing upward.

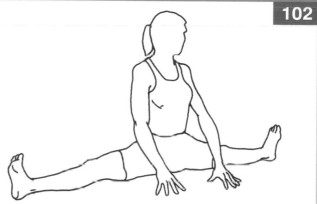

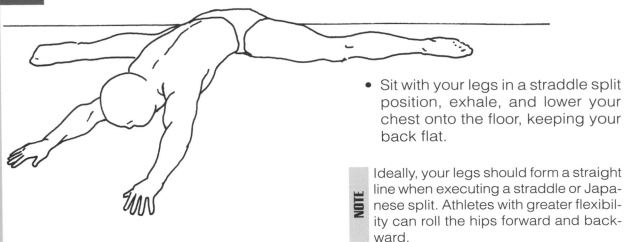

- Sit with your legs in a straddle split position, exhale, and lower your chest onto the floor, keeping your back flat.

NOTE Ideally, your legs should form a straight line when executing a straddle or Japanese split. Athletes with greater flexibility can roll the hips forward and backward.

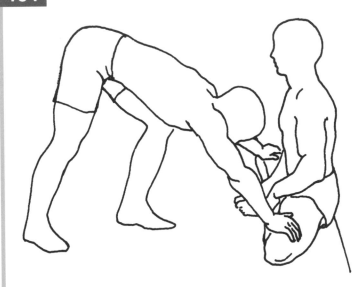

- Sit on the floor with your buttocks against a wall, back straight, legs flexed and spread, and heels touching each other.
- Grasp your feet or ankles and pull them as close to your groin as possible.
- Exhale as your partner assists in lowering your legs to the floor.

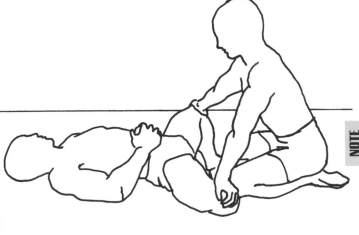

- Lie on your back and flex your knees, bringing the soles of your feet together as you pull them toward your groin.
- Exhale as your partner pushes your legs to the floor.

NOTE Be sure to communicate with your partner.

- Lie on your back; flex and spread your legs with the soles of your feet together and resting against the wall.
- Exhale as your partner pushes your legs to the floor.

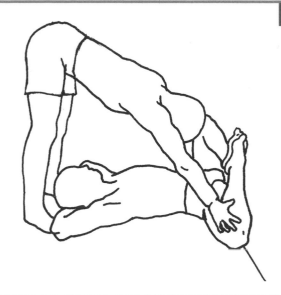

- Lie on your back with your legs raised and together and your buttocks several inches from a wall. Spread your legs as wide as possible.
- Exhale as your partner spreads your legs farther apart while keeping both legs straight.

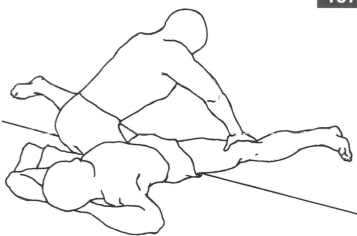

- Lie on your back with both legs raised vertically and spread.
- Your partner grasps both ankles as you lower your legs and assists in spreading them farther apart.

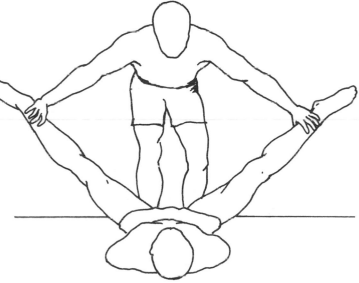

109

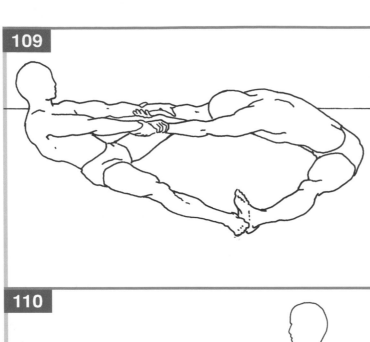

- Sit on the floor with your legs spread. Your partner assumes the same position with feet braced against yours. Lean forward and grasp each other's wrists.
- Exhale; keeping your legs straight, extend your upper torso and bend forward at the hips as your partner leans backward and pulls on your wrists.

110

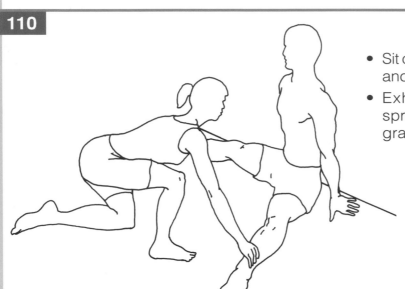

- Sit on the floor with your legs spread and your buttocks against a wall.
- Exhale as your partner gently spreads your legs farther apart by grasping your ankles or shins.

111

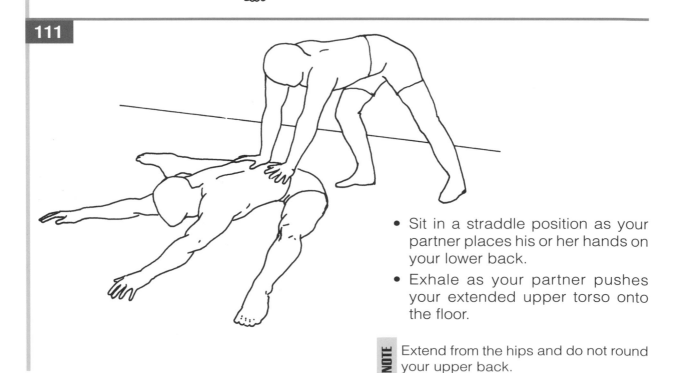

- Sit in a straddle position as your partner places his or her hands on your lower back.
- Exhale as your partner pushes your extended upper torso onto the floor.

NOTE Extend from the hips and do not round your upper back.

- Kneel with your toes pointing out to the sides. Rest your elbows on the floor.
- Exhale, spread your knees, and attempt to lower your chest to the floor.
- Your partner kneels at your side or directly behind you and places his hands on your buttocks and upper back.
- Exhale as your partner pushes to spread your knees and lower your pubic bone to the floor.

 NOTE Be sure to communicate with your partner. This is a very intense stretch.

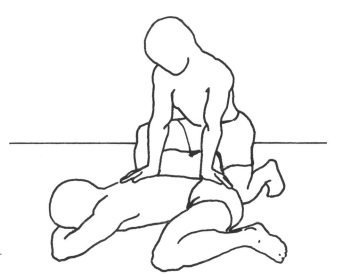

- Kneel on all fours with your toes pointing backward.
- Your partner stands on your right side, sliding his right leg between your legs, and hooks your right ankle or leg (grapevine). He reaches across your lower back and grasps your left knee.
- Your partner pulls your left knee from the floor and rolls to his right, with you following. When the roll is completed, your partner is on his back with your back and buttocks on his stomach and your legs spread. If necessary, your partner can hook his left foot over your right foot.
- Exhale as your partner gently pulls your legs apart.

 Make sure your left knee is flexed to avoid excessive stress on the medial part.

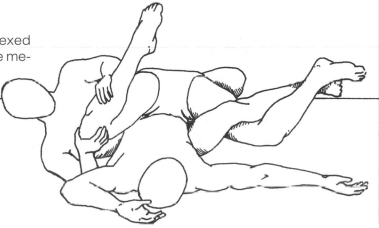

114

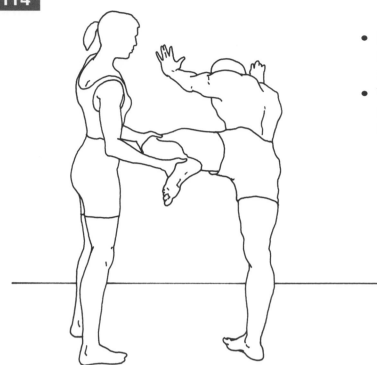

- Stand with your hands resting on a wall. Inhale, flex one knee, and raise it sideways.
- Your partner grasps your ankle and knee. Exhale as your partner raises your leg farther.

115

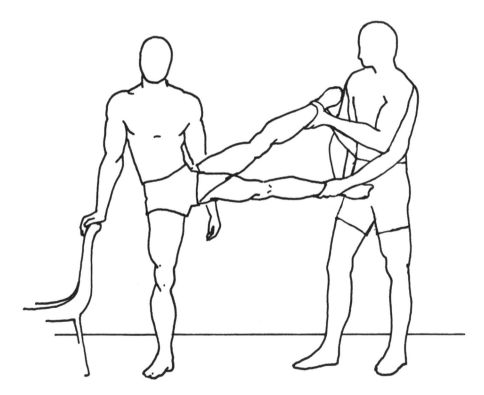

- Stand holding onto a surface for balance and raise one leg sideways.
- Your partner grasps your heel and lower leg above your ankle. Exhale as your partner raises your leg.

 NOTE Concentrate on preventing your buttocks from protruding during this stretch. Be sure to communicate with your partner.

- Stand facing your partner and place your leg on your partner's shoulder.
- Turn your hip so your feet face away from your partner and exhale as your partner steps away from you.

NOTE This is a very advanced partner stretch used in the martial arts; it is not necessary for most athletes. Be sure to communicate with your partner.

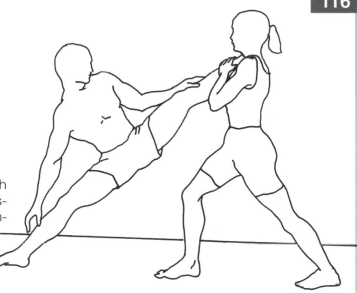

- Stand holding a pair of lightweight dumbbells with your legs parallel and feet shoulder-width apart.
- Step forward with one foot and lower your body until your back knee rests on the floor.
- Exhale and return to the starting position.

NOTE Start with a light weight, and do not lift the heel of your leading foot or allow your knee to go past your toes. The angle of your flexed knee should be no greater than 90 degrees.

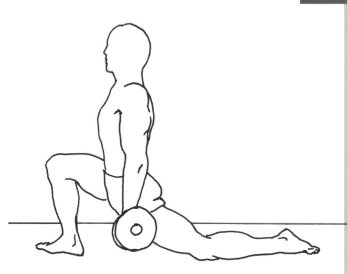

- Stand holding a lightweight barbell across your shoulders. Start with your legs parallel and feet shoulder-width apart.
- Step forward with one foot and lower your body until your back knee rests on the floor.
- Exhale and return to the starting position.

NOTE Be sure the angle of your flexed knee does not exceed 90 degrees.

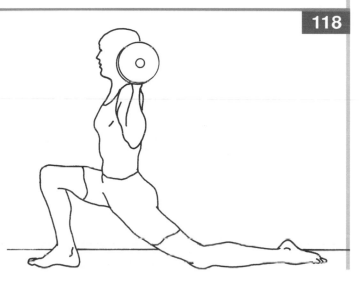

QUADRICEPS

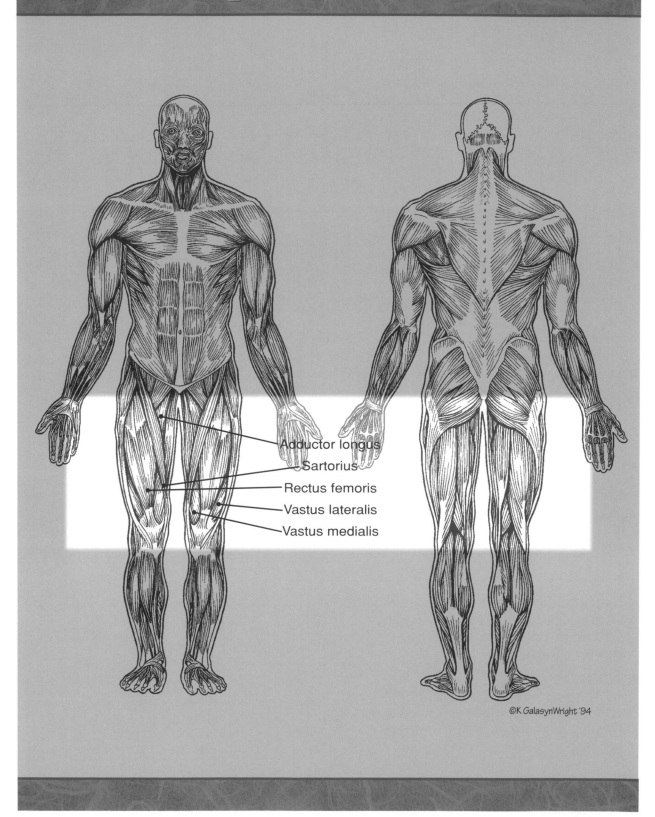

Adductor longus

Sartorius

Rectus femoris

Vastus lateralis

Vastus medialis

©K GalasynWright '94

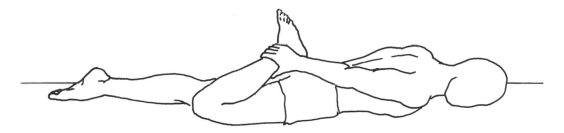

- Lie face down, flex one knee, and raise your heel toward your buttocks.
- Exhale, grasp your raised ankle, and pull your heel toward your buttocks without overcompressing the knee.

 NOTE To maximize the stretch, make sure the medial sides of your legs touch each other and your pelvis rotates backward (visualize pulling your tailbone between your legs).

 Do not arch your lower back or twist your pelvis.

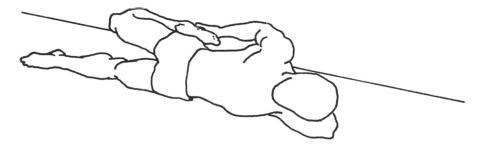

- Lie on your side, flex one knee, and raise your heel toward your buttocks.
- Exhale, grasp your raised ankle, and pull your heel toward your buttocks without overcompressing the knee.

 NOTE Io maximize the stretch, make sure the medial sides of your legs touch each other and your pelvis rotates backward (visualize pulling your tailbone between your legs).

 Do not arch your lower back or twist your pelvis.

121

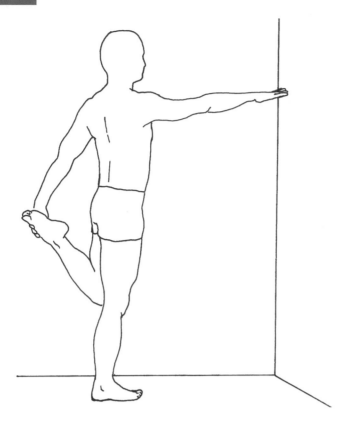

- Stand holding onto something for balance. Flex one knee and raise your heel to your buttocks.
- Slightly flex your supporting leg, exhale, and grasp your raised foot with one hand.
- Inhale and slowly pull your heel toward your buttocks without overcompressing the knee.

NOTE To maximize the stretch, make sure the medial sides of your legs touch each other and your pelvis rotates backward (visualize pulling your tailbone between your legs).

 Do not arch your lower back or twist your pelvis.

122

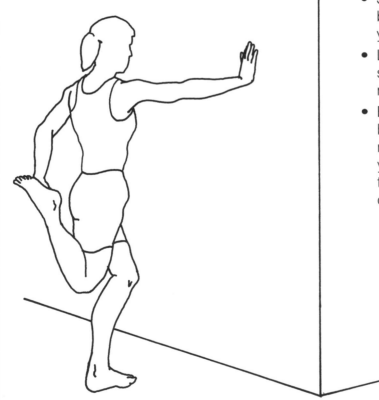

- Stand holding onto something for balance. Flex one knee and raise your heel to your buttocks.
- Lean forward, slightly flex your supporting leg, and grasp your raised foot with the opposite hand.
- Exhale, pull your heel toward your buttocks, and crisscross the raised knee behind the knee of your supporting leg. Pull your heel toward your buttocks without overcompressing the knee.

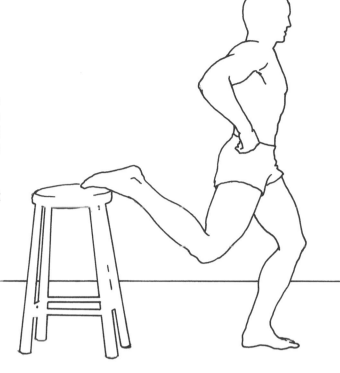

- Stand with the top of one foot resting on a chair behind you.
- Inhale and slowly flex your front knee.

NOTE To maximize the stretch, make sure the medial sides of your legs touch each other and your pelvis rotates backward (visualize pulling your tailbone between your legs).

⚠ Do not arch your lower back or twist your pelvis.

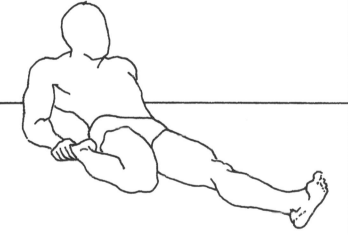

- Sit on the floor and bend your right leg behind you so that the inside of the knee and thigh are on the floor and the foot points along the line of the lower leg in a relaxed position.
- Exhale; lean diagonally back onto the forearm and elbow opposite your rear leg without arching your lower back. Continue leaning backward until you are flat on your back.

NOTE To increase the stretch, contract the gluteals and lift the hip off the floor.

⚠ Do not let the foot of your rear leg flare out to the side. To guard against excessive stress on the lumbar spine, keep your forward leg in a slightly flexed position.

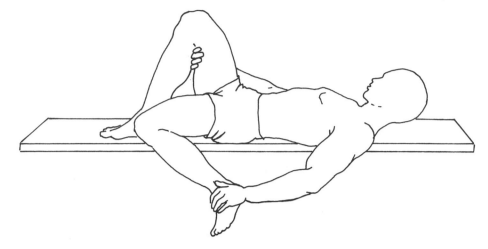

- Lie on your back on the edge of a table. Flex your inside leg and slide it toward your buttocks to help in anchoring your hips. Grasp the underside of the flexed knee with your inside hand.
- Exhale, lower your outside leg off the table at the hip, grasp the ankle or foot with your outside hand, and pull your heel toward your buttocks.

 NOTE You should feel the stretch in the middle to upper thigh.

 To protect your lower back, lift your head and contract your abdominal muscles.

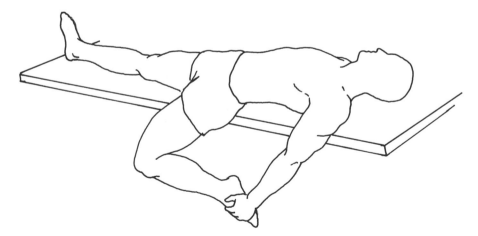

- Lie on your back on the edge of a table. Exhale, lower your outside leg off the table at the hip, and grasp your ankle or foot with your outside hand.
- Exhale and pull your heel toward your buttocks.

 NOTE You should feel the stretch in the middle to upper thigh.

 To protect your lower back, lift your head and contract your abdominal muscles.

- Squat with both hands on the floor for support and one leg resting on the floor.
- Grasp your rear foot and pull your heel toward your buttocks. Be careful to maintain parallel alignment of the hips, knees, and feet of both legs.

 Use a sturdy chair for balance if needed.

 Do not arch your lower back, twist your pelvis, or place too much weight on the knee resting on the floor.

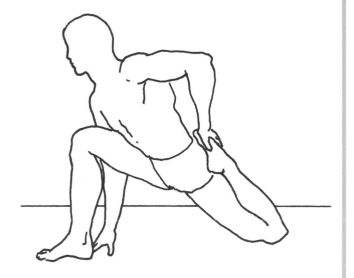

- Stand parallel to a bench or table, holding onto it for balance.
- Raise the leg closest to the bench and rest it on the surface. Flex your leg to your buttocks.
- Exhale and pull your heel toward your buttocks.

NOTE Use a rope or towel hooked around the ankle if needed.

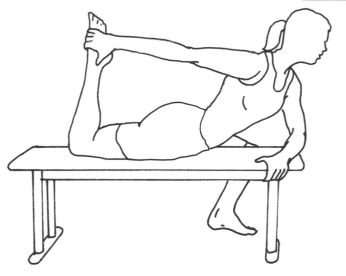

- Sit on the edge of an elevated platform (a pile of mats or a bed) about three feet above the floor with both legs hanging over the edge at the knee.
- Assume a split position with your back leg resting on the platform.
- Exhale, flex the rear knee, and slowly pull your heel toward your head.

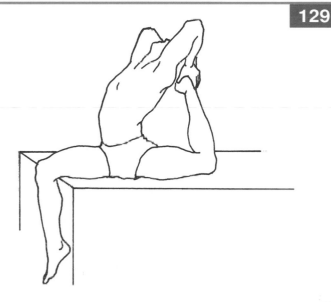

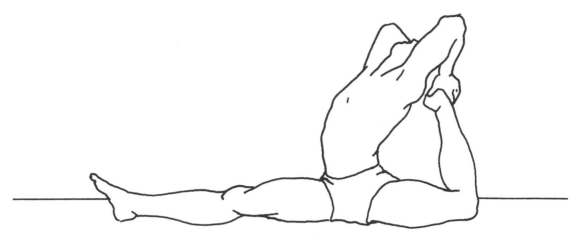

- Kneeling with both legs together and your hands at your sides, lift one knee and place your foot slightly in front for support.
- Bend at the hips, lower your upper torso onto your front thigh, and place your hands slightly in front of your front foot for support.
- Exhale, slide your front foot forward, and straighten your rear leg as you extend into the split position. Flex your rear leg and slowly pull your rear foot toward your head.

NOTE You should also feel this stretch in your hamstrings. To maximize the stretch, both legs must be straight, the hips squared (facing front, not twisted sideways), and the buttocks flat on the floor.

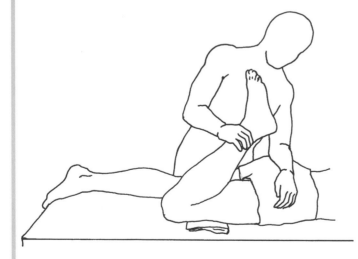

- Lie face down with one leg flexed toward your buttocks.
- Your partner anchors your buttocks or hips with one hand and grasps your ankle with the other.
- Exhale as your partner pushes your heel toward your buttocks without overcompressing the knee.

NOTE Place a cushion or folded towel under the stretched leg to reduce discomfort.

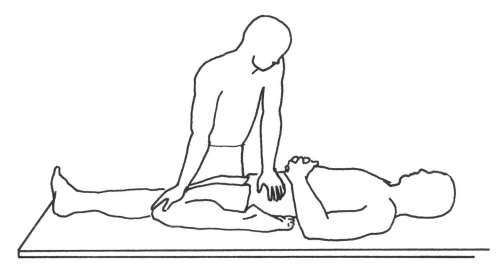

- Lie on a bench or table with your left leg flexed behind you so that the inside of your knee and thigh rest on the surface and your foot points toward your left shoulder.
- Your partner anchors your hip with one hand and your knee with the other.
- Exhale as your partner gently pushes down on your hip and knee.

NOTE To protect your knee, do not let the foot of your rear leg flare out to the side.

- Kneel with your toes pointing backward.
- Exhale and sit on the top of your heels.

⚠️ Make sure your buttocks sit on top of your heels and not between your feet. Do not do this stretch if you have knee problems.

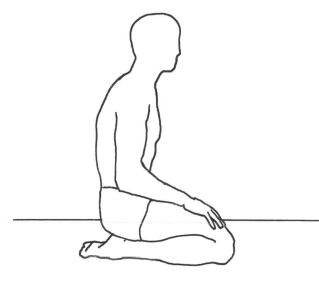

134

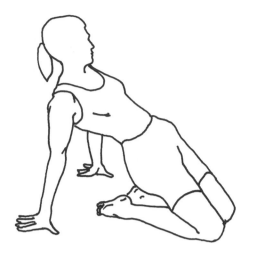

- Kneel with your knees together, buttocks on the floor, heels by the sides of your thighs, and toes pointing backward.

- Exhale and lean backward without letting your feet flare out to the sides.

⚠️ Do not arch your back. Instead, contract your gluteals and rotate your pelvis backward. Do not allow your knees to rise off the floor or spread apart.

135

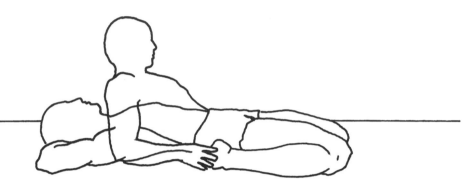

- Kneel with your knees together, buttocks on the floor, heels by the sides of your thighs, and toes pointing backward.

- Exhale as you continue leaning backward until you are flat on your back. Do not let your feet flare out to the sides.

NOTE Do not arch your back. Instead, contract your gluteals and rotate your pelvis backward. Do not allow your feet to flare out to the side or your knees to rise off the floor or spread apart.

HIPS AND GLUTEALS

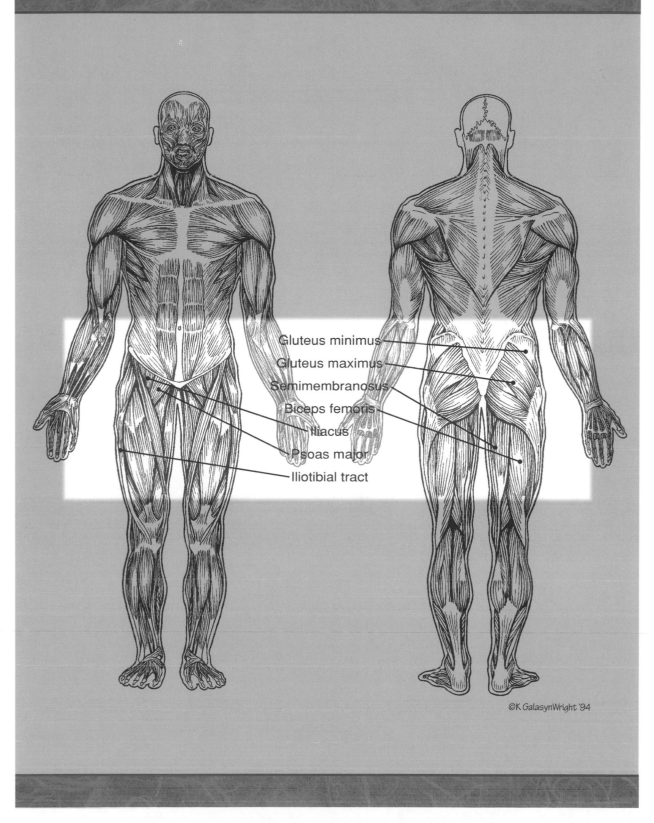

Gluteus minimus

Gluteus maximus

Semimembranosus

Biceps femoris

Iliacus

Psoas major

Iliotibial tract

©K.GalasynWright '94

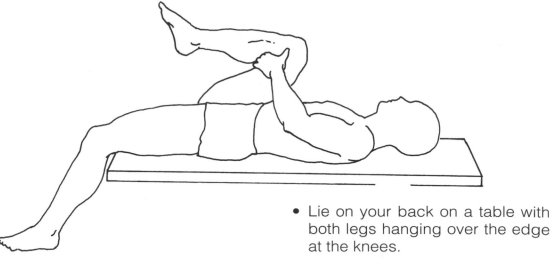

- Lie on your back on a table with both legs hanging over the edge at the knees.
- Inhale, flex one hip, and raise your knee toward your chest; interlock your hands behind the raised knee.
- Inhale and bring your knee to your chest as you keep the opposite leg hanging over the edge.

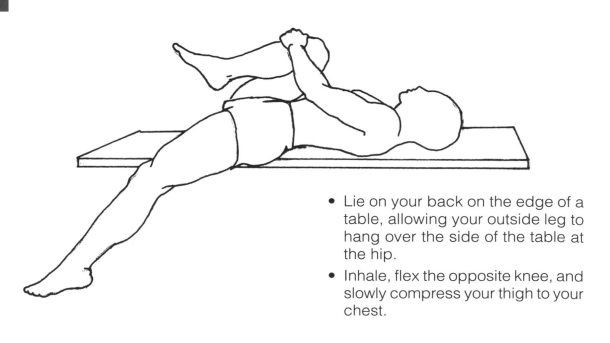

- Lie on your back on the edge of a table, allowing your outside leg to hang over the side of the table at the hip.
- Inhale, flex the opposite knee, and slowly compress your thigh to your chest.

- Stand with your legs spread about two feet apart. Flex one knee, lower your body, and place the opposite knee on the floor.
- Roll your back foot under so that the top of the instep rests on the floor.
- Place your hands on your hips (or one hand on your forward knee and one hand on your buttocks) and keep your front knee bent at a 90-degree angle.
- Exhale and push the front of the hip of your back leg toward the floor.

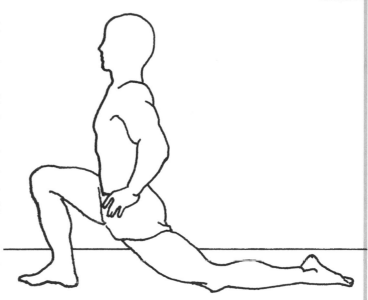

- Stand parallel to a three-foot-high (one-meter-high) bench or table.
- Flex your knees and place your inside hand on the face of the bench for balance.
- Swing the leg closest to the bench back into a split position with your leg on the bench.
- Exhale and push down (press up) on the bench with the supporting hand. Keep your hips squared and turned under.

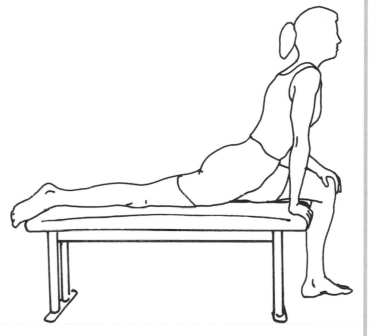

140

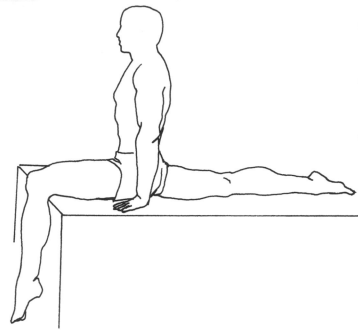

- Sit on an elevated platform (a pile of mats or a bed) about three feet (one meter) above the floor.
- Swing one leg back, assuming a split position with the leg resting on the platform.
- Exhale and push down (press up) on the platform with both hands. Keep your hips squared and turned under.

141

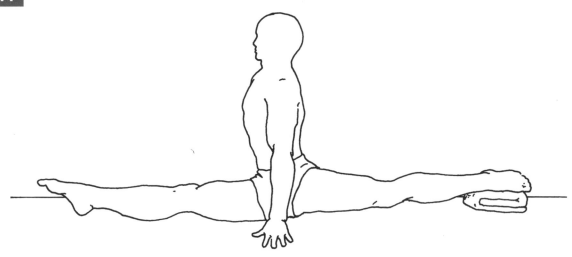

- Kneeling with both legs together and your hands at your sides, lift one knee and place your foot slightly in front for support.
- Exhale, bend at the hips, lower your upper torso onto your front thigh, and place your hands slightly in front of your front foot.
- Slide your front foot forward and straighten your rear leg and rest it on a folded mat as you extend into the split position.

NOTE For aesthetic reasons, some advocate a slight turnout of the rear hip when doing the splits. However, due to tight hip flexors or improper training, this turnout can be too extreme for many individuals.

- Lie face down with one knee flexed.
- Your partner places one hand under your knee (on front of the thigh) and the other slightly above or on the side of your buttocks.
- Contract your gluteals as your partner anchors your abdomen to the table or floor with one hand and gently lifts your leg higher with the other.

⚠ This exercise creates an intense stretch. Be sure to communicate with your partner.

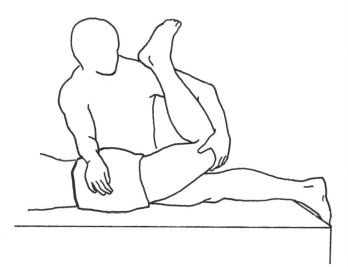

- Lie on your back on the edge of a table.
- Exhale, lower your outside leg off the table at the hip, and grasp your ankle or foot with your outside hand, pulling your heel toward your buttocks.
- Your partner stands at your side with one hand on your left knee and the other on your right hip. Exhale as your partner gently presses on your hip and knee.

⚠ To protect your lower back, lift your head and contract your abdominal muscles.

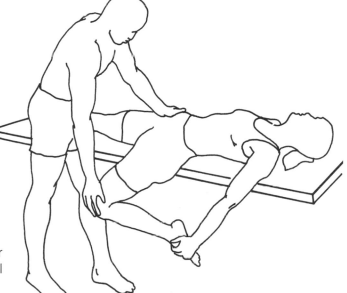

144

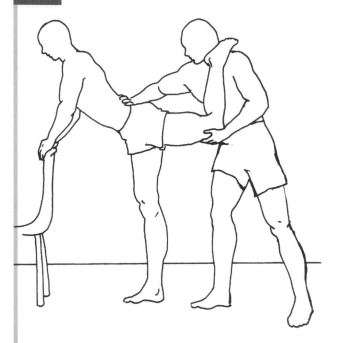

- Stand with one foot turned slightly outward. Hold onto a surface for balance.
- Exhale, bend at your hips, and flex the raised knee.
- Your partner places one hand under your raised knee and the other above your buttocks.
- Inhale as your partner anchors your body with one hand and lifts your raised leg with the other.

⚠️ Hyperextending the back when performing an arabesque can cause injury. Spread the extension through all the joints of the spine instead of forcing it all to the bottom of the spine.

145

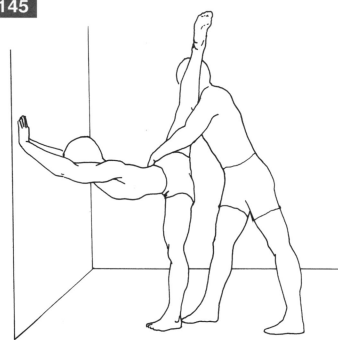

- Stand with one foot turned slightly outward. Hold onto a surface for balance.
- Exhale, bend at your hips, and raise your leg behind you, keeping it straight.
- Your partner stands behind you, rests your raised thigh on his shoulder, reaches over your raised leg, interlocks his fingers, and places his hands on your upper buttocks.
- Inhale as your partner anchors your body with one hand and raises your extended thigh up and forward with his shoulder.

146

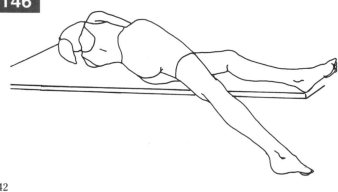

- Lie on your side on the edge of a table with your legs extended.
- Exhale and extend and adduct one leg so it hangs over the edge.

NOTE You should feel this stretch in the iliotibial band.

- Lie on your back with your legs extended.
- Flex one knee, raise it to your chest, and grasp it with the opposite hand.
- Exhale and pull your knee across your body to the floor, keeping your elbows, head, and shoulders flat on the floor.

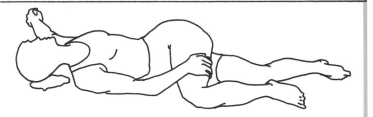

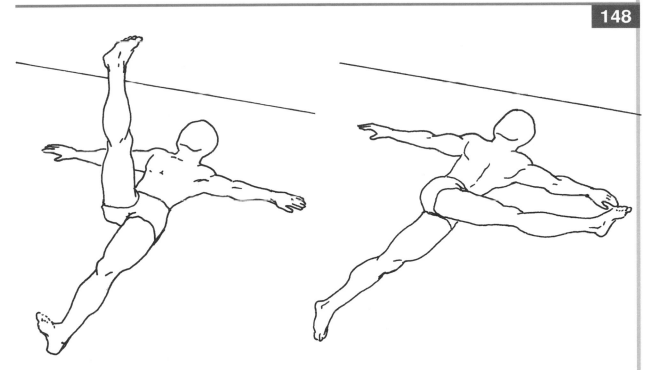

- Lie on your back with one leg raised and straight and your arms out to your sides.
- Exhale and lower your raised leg toward the opposite hand, keeping your elbows, head, and shoulders flat on the floor.

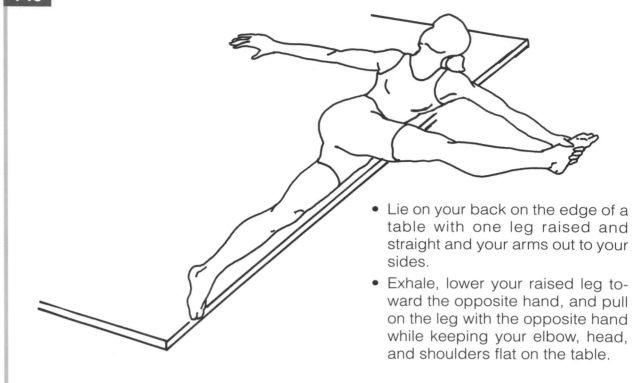

149

- Lie on your back on the edge of a table with one leg raised and straight and your arms out to your sides.
- Exhale, lower your raised leg toward the opposite hand, and pull on the leg with the opposite hand while keeping your elbow, head, and shoulders flat on the table.

150

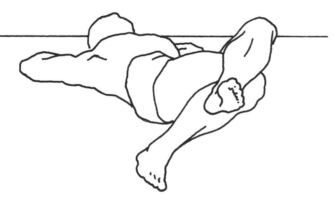

- Lie on your back, knees flexed, and hands interlocked under your head.
- Lift your left leg and hook it over your right leg.
- Exhale and use your left leg to force the inside of your right leg to the floor, keeping your elbows, head, and shoulders flat on the floor.

151

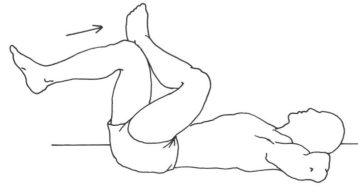

- Lie on your back with your left leg crossed over your right knee.
- Exhale and flex your right knee, lifting your right foot off the floor, and let it slowly push your left foot toward your face, keeping your head, shoulders, and back flat on the floor.

- Lie on your back with your knees flexed and arms out to the sides.
- Exhale and lower both legs to the floor on the same side, keeping your elbows, head, and shoulders flat on the floor.

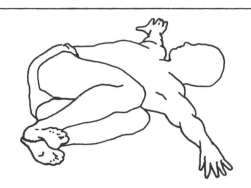

- Lie on your back with your legs raised straight and arms out to the sides.
- Exhale and lower both legs to the floor on the same side, keeping your elbows, head, and shoulders flat on the floor.

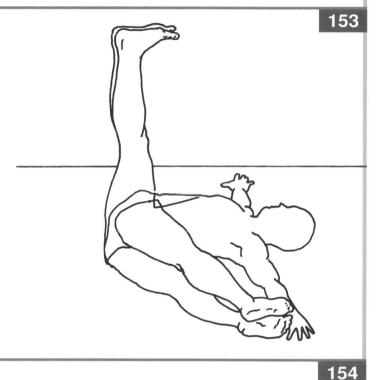

- Sit on a chair with one leg flexed and your heel resting on the chair edge. Interlock both hands and grasp your raised knee.
- Exhale and pull your knee to and across your body as your heel remains flat on the chair.

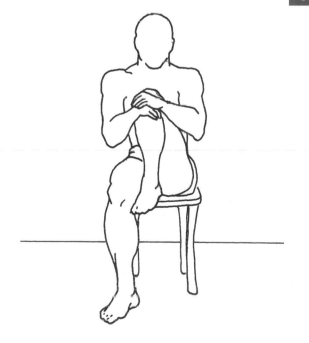

155

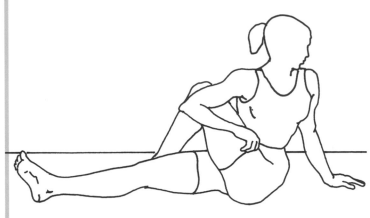

- Sit on the floor with your hands behind your hips and your legs extended.
- Cross your left foot over your right leg and slide your heel toward your buttocks. Place your right elbow on the outside of your left knee.
- Exhale and look over your left shoulder while turning your trunk and gently pushing on your knee with your right elbow.

156

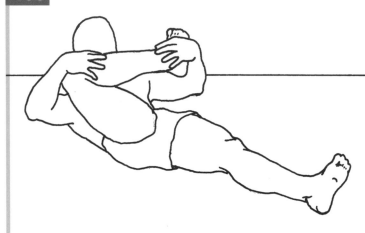

- Lie on the floor, flex one leg, and slide the heel toward your buttocks.
- Grasp your knee with the same-side hand and your ankle with the opposite hand.
- Exhale and pull your foot to the opposite shoulder, keeping your shoulders and back flat on the floor.

157

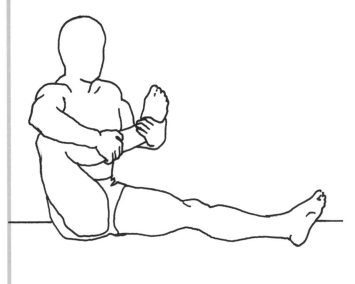

- Sit on the floor with your back against a wall. Flex one leg and slide your heel toward your buttocks.
- Hook your knee with the same-side elbow and grasp your ankle with the opposite hand.
- Exhale and pull your foot to the opposite shoulder.

 NOTE Keep your back straight and upright.

- Sit on the floor and cross one knee over the over.
- Exhale and lean forward.

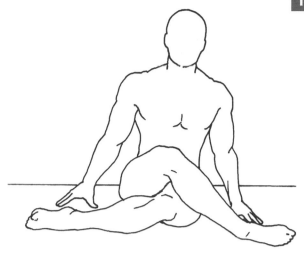

- Sit on a chair or on the floor with one leg crossed over the opposite knee.
- Place your hand on the medial part of your knee, exhale, and lean forward.

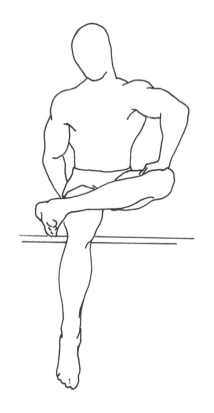

- Sit on the floor and flex your left knee so that your left foot points to your right.
- Cross your right leg over your left leg and place your right foot flat on the floor.
- Exhale, bend your upper torso forward, and place your head on your bottom knee.

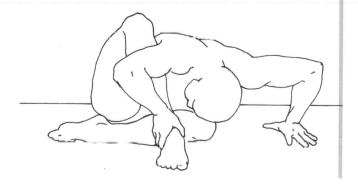

161

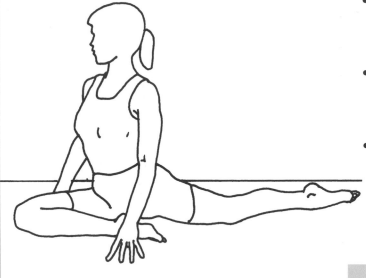

- Sit on the floor with both legs straight and your palms flat on the floor by your hips with your fingers pointing toward your feet.
- Flex your right knee and place your right foot on the floor so that the heel touches your left knee. Do not let your right leg rise off the floor.
- Inhale and extend your left leg behind you. The front of your left thigh, kneecap, shin, instep, and the upper part of your toes should rest on the floor. Exhale and push your right hip into the floor.

NOTE Intensify this stretch by moving your right foot away from the thigh until your upper and lower legs form a right angle.

162

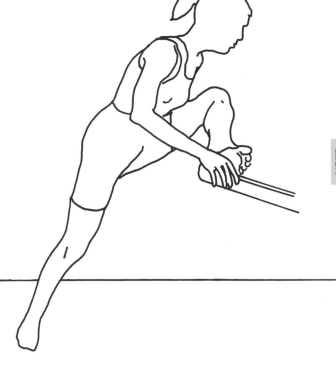

- Stand an arm's length from a sturdy hip-height surface. Hold onto the surface.
- Inhale, flex one knee, move your pelvis forward, and place your outer thigh, calf, and ankle on the surface of the bench. Exhale and lean forward.

NOTE Use a padded bench or a folded towel to reduce discomfort.

- Sitting on the floor, flex your right knee and place your right foot as high as possible on your left thigh with the sole of your foot turned up.
- Exhale, flex your left knee, and place it as high as possible on your right thigh with the sole turned up and without forcing the stretch.

 This stretch, called the Padma or Lotus, is one of the most important meditative poses in yoga.

 This stretch is not recommended for individuals with knee problems.

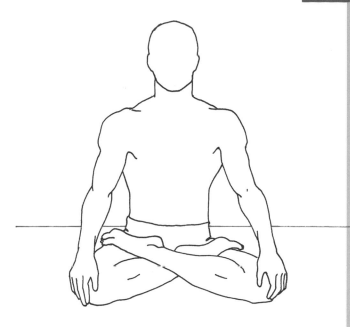

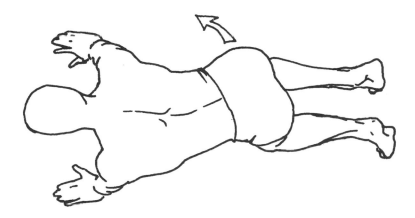

- Kneel on all fours.
- Exhale, flex one arm, and rotate your hip out to that side.

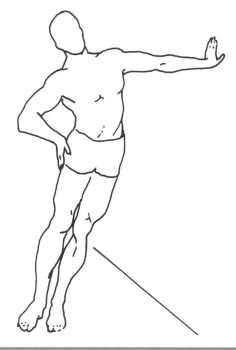

165

- Stand slightly more than an arm's length from a wall.
- Place one hand on the wall and the heel of your other hand on the back of your hip joint.
- Exhale; keeping your legs straight, contract your buttocks and rotate your hips slightly forward and in toward the wall.

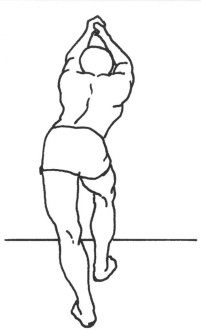

166

- Stand slightly more than an arm's length from a wall.
- Bend one leg forward and lean against the wall without losing the straight line of your head, neck, spine, pelvis, rear leg, and ankle.
- Keep the heel of your rear leg flat and parallel to your hips as you rotate the hip outward.

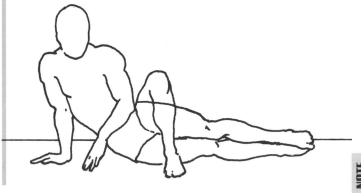

167

- Lie on your side with your knees and hips extended in a straight line with your torso.
- Exhale and push up to a resting position on your hip, placing your arm directly under your shoulder and bearing weight on your extended arm and hand.

NOTE You may have to place your opposite foot on the floor to stabilize your pelvis.

150

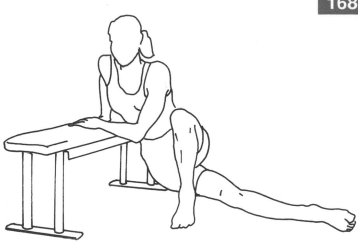

- Sit on the floor with your arms straight and hands resting on the surface of a bench. Extend your legs laterally.
- Exhale and turn your body laterally, crossing your left leg over your right knee and placing your left foot on the floor.
- Exhale, bend the supporting arms, and allow the extended leg to slide away from the bench while attempting to lower your hip to the floor.

 This stretch is used by dancers to correct a snapping hip.

Do not do this stretch if you have a history of lateral ligament injury to the knee.

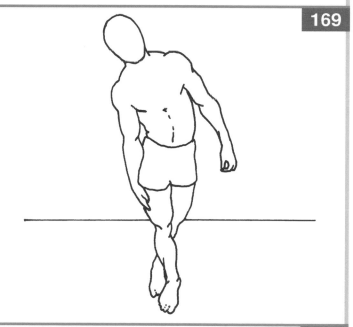

- Stand with your hands at your sides and extend and adduct your left leg as far as possible.
- Exhale and flex your trunk laterally toward your right side, keeping your hands by your hips.

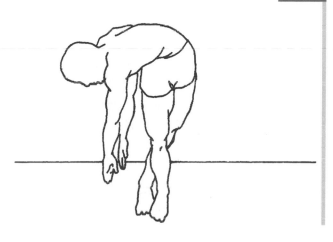

- Stand with your hands at your sides and extend and adduct your left leg as far as possible.
- Exhale and flex your torso laterally toward your right side. Try to touch the heel of your left leg with both hands.
- Exhale, round your upper torso, and return to the starting position.

This is a severe stretch since it incorporates both spinal flexion and rotation.

171

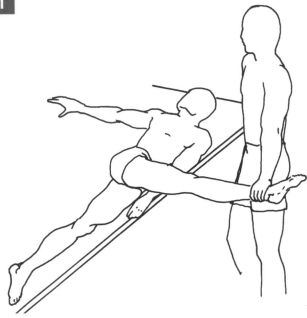

- Lie on your back on the edge of a table with one leg raised and straight and your arms out to the sides.
- Lower your raised leg to the opposite side for your partner to grasp.
- Exhale as your partner pushes down on your hanging leg, keeping your head and shoulders flat on the table.

NOTE Be sure to communicate with your partner.

172

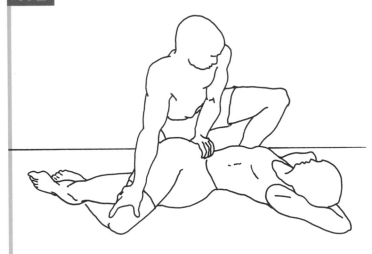

- Lie on your back with your knees flexed and your hands interlocked beneath your head.
- Hook your right leg over your left leg.
- Your partner anchors your body with one hand on your hip and the other on your right knee.
- Exhale as your partner gently pushes your right leg to the floor, keeping your elbows, head, and shoulders flat on the floor.

173

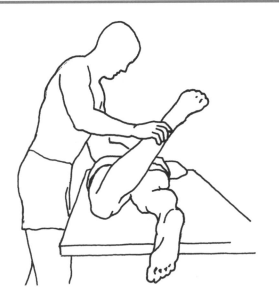

- Lie face down on a table with your body extended. Flex the leg nearest the table edge.
- Your partner anchors your body with one hand and grasps the ankle of the flexed leg with the other. Exhale as your partner pushes your leg toward the opposite side.

- Lie on your back and raise one leg so your thigh is nearly vertical and your knee is flexed.
- Exhale and move the foot of the raised leg in toward your body.
- Your partner holds your knee and ankle on the side to be stretched.
- Exhale as your partner moves your foot toward your body.

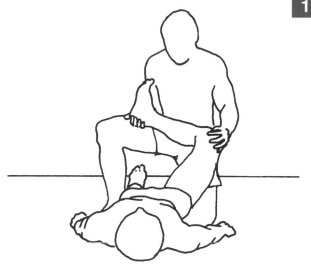

175

- Stand with your right side against a wall, flex your left knee, and raise your right foot.
- Your partner stands in front of you and grasps your raised leg in a flexed position.
- Exhale as your partner pushes your leg, bending your knee even farther.

NOTE This is an advanced stretch used in the martial arts.

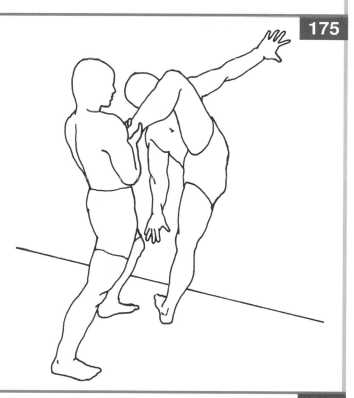

176

- Lie face down on a table and flex the leg nearest the table edge.
- Your partner anchors your body with one hand and grasps your flexed lower leg with the other.
- Exhale as your partner pulls your leg away from your body.

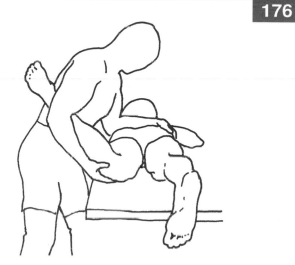

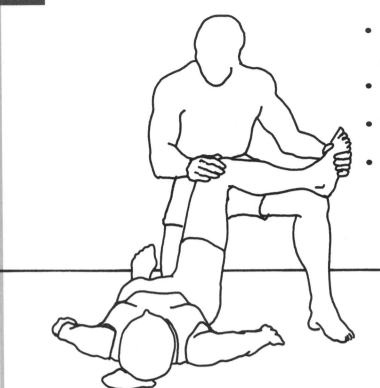

- Lie on your back and raise one leg so the thigh is nearly vertical and the knee is flexed.
- Exhale and slowly move your raised foot away from your body.
- Your partner holds the knee and ankle of the side to be stretched.
- Exhale as your partner slowly moves your raised foot away from your body.

LOWER TORSO

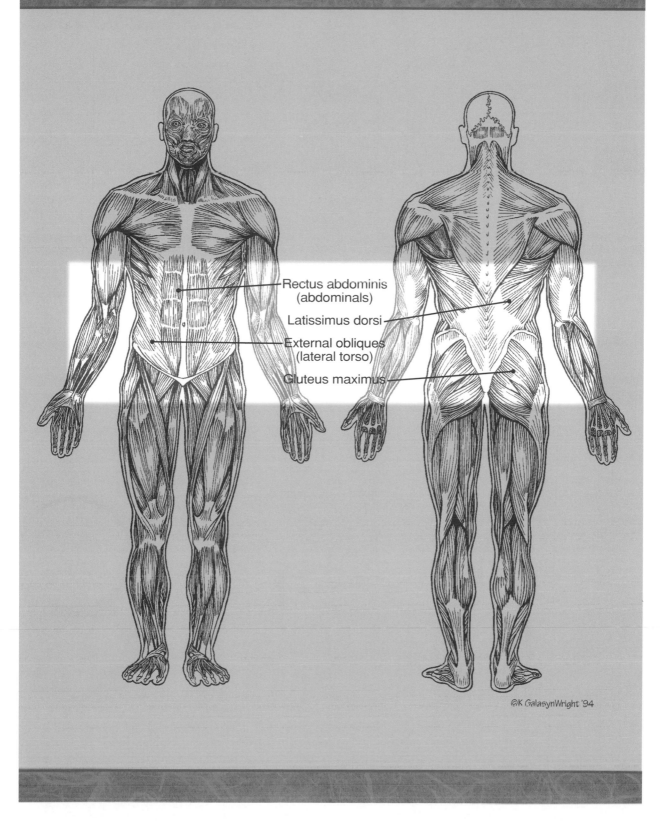

Rectus abdominis
(abdominals)

Latissimus dorsi

External obliques
(lateral torso)

Gluteus maximus

©K GalasynWright '94

178

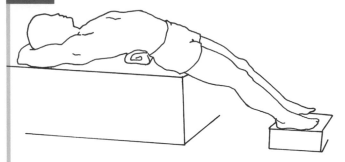

- Lie on a bed on your back.
- Exhale and slide your lower torso so it hangs over the edge.

 Do not do this stretch if you have lordosis.

179

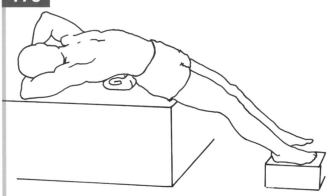

- Lie on a bed on your back with your lower torso hanging over the edge.
- Exhale and lift one elbow off the surface.

 Do not do this stretch if you have lordosis.

180

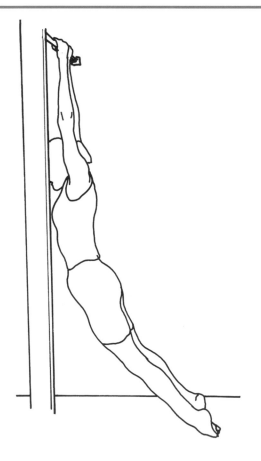

- Stand facing a chin-up bar that is lower than head height. Grasp it with both hands almost touching in an overgrip.
- Exhale, keep your arms straight, and hang from the chin-up bar with your body arched.

NOTE You can achieve the same effect by hanging from the edge of a baseball dugout.

- Lie face down on the floor with your body extended.
- Place your palms on the floor by your hips with your fingers pointing forward.
- Exhale, press down on the floor, raise your head and trunk, and arch your back while contracting the gluteals to prevent excessive compression of your lower back.

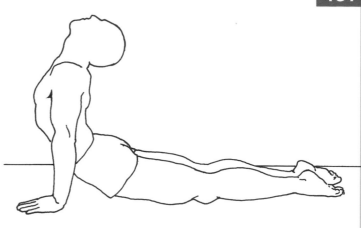

- Kneel on the floor with your legs slightly apart and parallel and your toes pointing backward.
- Place your palms on your upper hips, arch your back, contract your buttocks, and push your hips forward.
- Exhale, continue to arch your back, drop your head backward, and gradually slide your hands onto your heels.

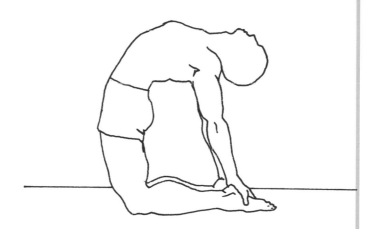

- Stand with your legs spread about three feet (one meter) apart and your hands on your buttocks.
- Arch your back, contract your buttocks, and push your hips forward.
- Exhale, continue arching your back, drop your head backward, open your mouth, and gradually slide your hands below your buttocks.

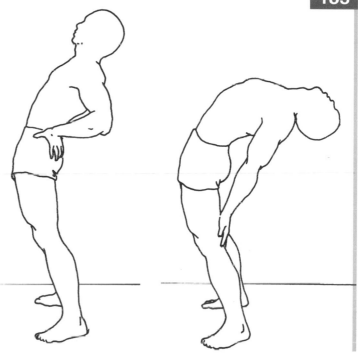

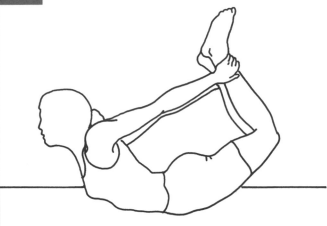

- Lie face down on the floor, flex your knees, and move your heels toward your hips.
- Inhale, grasp both ankles, contract your buttocks, and lift your chest and knees off the floor.

NOTE This common asana in yoga can be intensified by either resting the soles of the feet on the back of the head or fully extending into a vertical position.

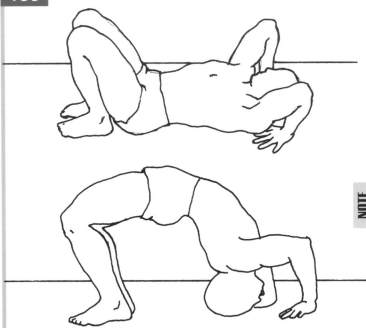

- Lie on your back with your heels close to your hips, the palms of your hands on the floor by your neck (under the shoulders), and your fingers pointing toward your feet.
- Inhale, raise your trunk, and rest your forehead on the floor.

NOTE This exercise is essential for practitioners of judo and wrestling.

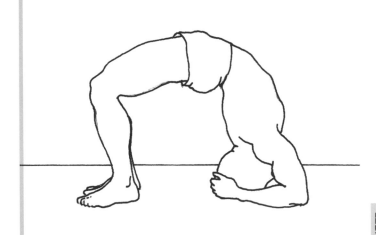

- Lie on your back with your heels close to your hips, the palms of your hands on the floor by your neck (under the shoulders), and your fingers pointing toward your feet.
- Inhale, raise your trunk, rest your forehead on the floor, raise one arm at a time, and place your forearms on the floor.

NOTE This exercise is essential for practitioners of judo and wrestling.

- Lie on your back with your heels close to your hips, the palms of your hands on the floor by your neck (under the shoulders), and your fingers pointing toward your feet.
- Exhale, extend your arms and legs, and raise your body into a full bridge with your wrists parallel to your shoulders.

NOTE This exercise is essential for gymnastics. You should also feel this stretch in the shoulders.

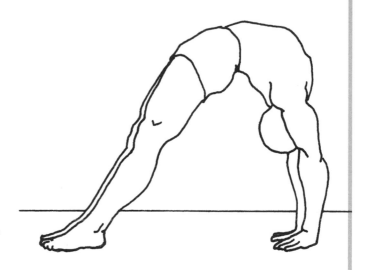

- Stand with your back about three feet (one meter) from a wall. Rest your hands on the wall at head height.
- Exhale and "walk" your hands down the wall. If necessary, use a spotter to provide assistance.
- Walk your hands up the wall to your starting position.

NOTE This is an excellent lead-up exercise for mastering the back walkover.

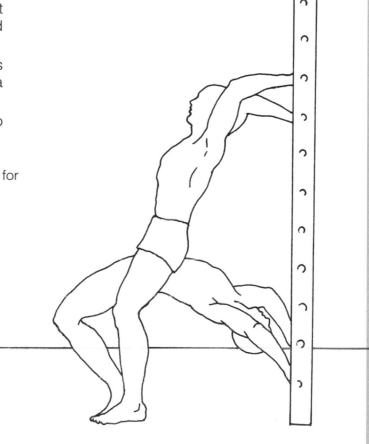

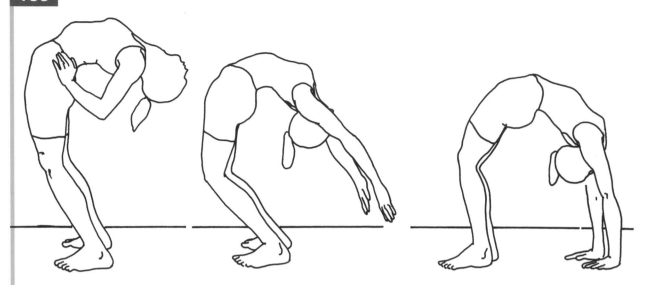

- Stand with your feet shoulder-width apart and your hands on your hips. Exhale, push your hips forward, and arch your back.
- Raise your arms overhead while continuing to arch backward. Place your hands on the floor, ending in a bridge position with your arms straight and no more than shoulder-width apart.
- Flex your arms and lower yourself onto your shoulders.

 If necessary, use a spotter for assistance and support.

 This exercise may be too advanced or dangerous for even some elite athletes.

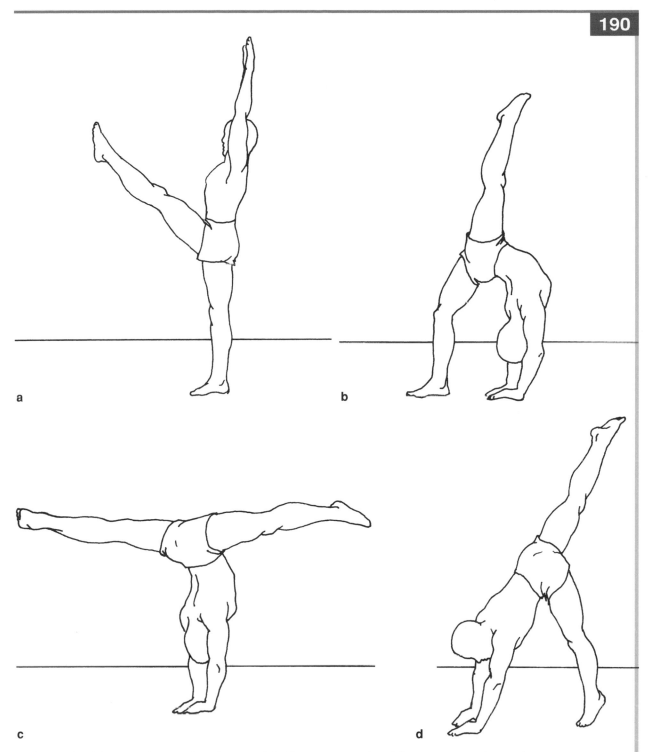

a

b

c

d

- Stand with one leg raised to a 90-degree angle, hips squared, and arms straight and vertical, elbows by your ears.
- Arch backward. Watch your hands contact the mat. Keep your arms straight and shoulder-width apart.
- Extend the ankle of your supporting foot and transfer your weight to your hands when your shoulders are directly over your hands. As your trailing leg leaves the floor, pass through a split position handstand, with your head between your arms and down.
- When your leading foot contacts the floor, your hands push off the floor.

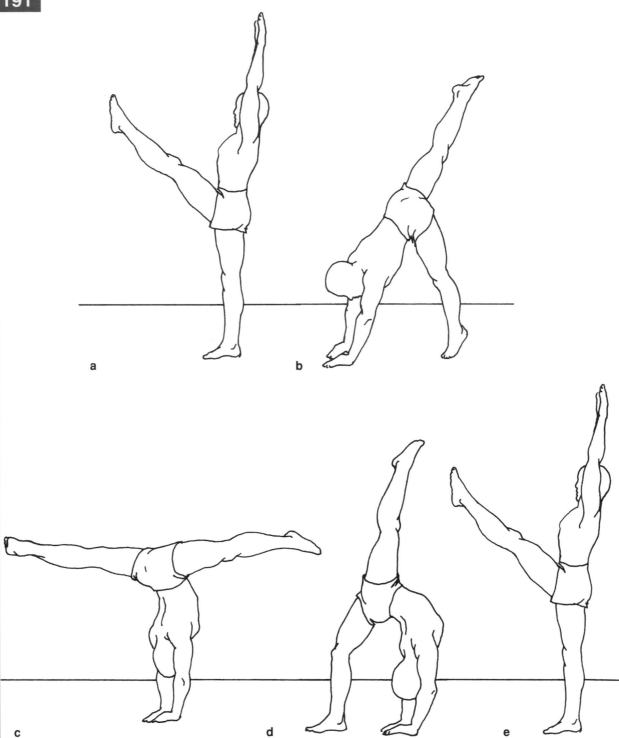

a   b

c   d   e

- Stand with one leg raised to a 90-degree angle, hips squared, and arms straight and vertical, elbows by your ears.
- Step forward, place your hands on the floor shoulder-width apart, and immediately push off with your supporting leg and arms.
- Continue to arch over and place your leading leg close to your hands.
- Push off with your hands, thrust your hips forward, straighten your supporting leg, and return to an upright position.

- Lie face down on the floor with your arms parallel and stretched forward.
- Your partner straddles your hips, facing your head, bends at the hips and knees, and grasps you between your shoulders and elbows.
- Inhale and contract your gluteals to prevent compression of your lower back as your partner lifts your upper torso off the floor.

 Communicate with your partner.

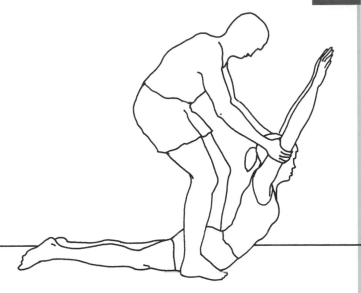

- Your partner straddles your hips, facing your feet, bends at the hips and knees, and grasps your lower legs.
- Exhale and contract your gluteals to prevent compression of your lower back as your partner lifts your thighs off the floor.

 This is an exceptionally intense stretch and should be done with caution.

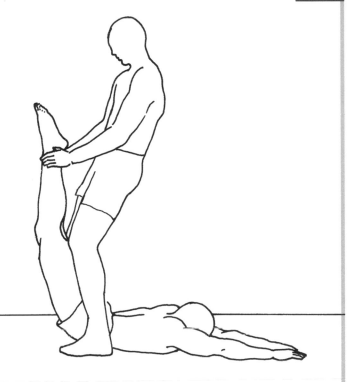

194

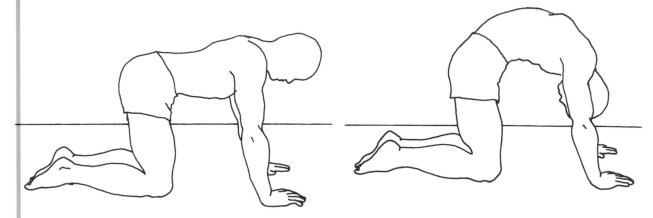

- Kneel on all fours with your toes pointing backward.
- Inhale, contract your abdominals, and round your back.
- Exhale, relax your abdominals, and return to the "flat back" position.

195

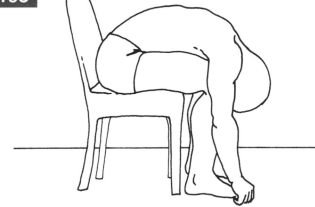

- Sit on a chair with your legs slightly separated.
- Exhale, extend your upper torso, bend at the hips, and lower your stomach between your thighs.

 NOTE Contracting your abdominals may help relax your lower back.

196

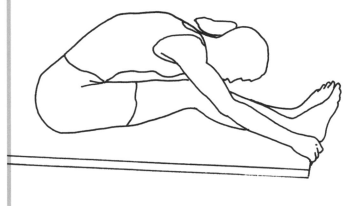

- Sit on a bed or bench with your knees flexed.
- Extend your upper torso, bend at the hips, and lower your stomach onto your thighs.
- Exhale and extend your legs.

 NOTE After a critical point, the sensation of this stretch may shift to the hamstrings. At this point, back off and hold the stretch. Contracting your abdominals may help relax your lower back.

- Lie on your back, flex your knees, and slide your feet toward your buttocks.
- Grasp behind your thighs to prevent hyperflexion of the knees.
- Exhale, pull your knees toward your chest and shoulders, and elevate your hips off the floor.
- Reextend your legs one at a time to prevent possible pain or spasm.

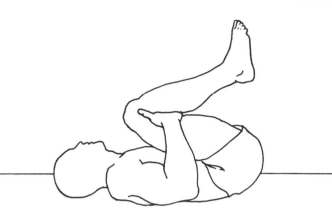

- Lie on your back, flex your knees, and slide your feet toward your buttocks.
- Your partner places one hand under your hamstrings and grasps your heels with the other.
- Exhale as your partner brings your thighs closer to your chest.
- Reextend your legs slowly one at a time to prevent possible pain or spasm.

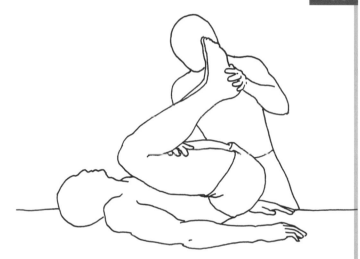

- Lie on your back with your arms by your hips, palms down.
- Exhale, push on the floor with your palms, and raise your legs in a squat position so your knees almost rest on your forehead. Support the weight of your hips with your hands.

 NOTE You should also feel this stretch in your posterior neck.

 Avoid excessive flexion of the neck.

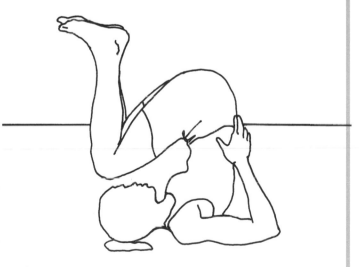

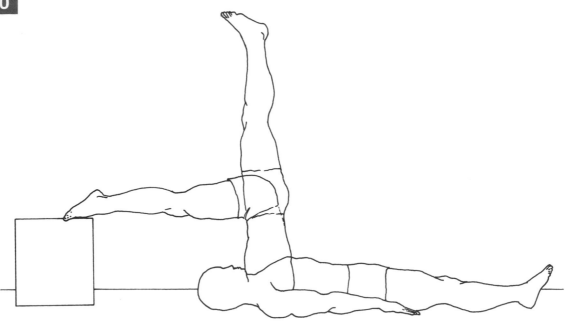

- Lie on your back with your arms by your hips, palms down.
- Inhale, push on the floor with your palms, and raise your legs to a vertical position.
- Exhale, keep your legs straight, and lower your feet onto a supporting surface about 12 to 24 inches (30 to 60 centimeters) off the floor.

NOTE You should also feel this stretch in your posterior neck.

 Avoid excessive flexion of the neck.

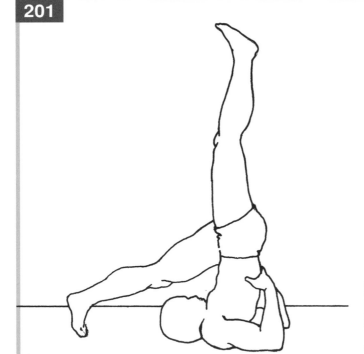

- Lie on your back with your arms by your hips, palms down.
- Inhale, push on the floor with your palms, raise your legs to a vertical position, and support your body with your hands placed on your lower back.
- Exhale, split your legs, and lower one foot to the floor while the other leg remains vertical. If you lack sufficient flexibility, only lower your leg to a horizontal position.

NOTE You should also feel this stretch in your posterior neck and the hamstrings of the leg contacting the floor.

 Avoid excessive flexion of the neck.

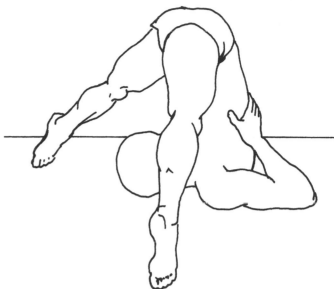

- Lie on your back with your arms by your hips, palms down.
- Inhale, push on the floor with your palms, raise your legs to a vertical position, and support your body with your hands placed on your lower back.
- Exhale, keep your legs straight and spread apart, and lower your feet to the floor.

 This exercise is essential for practitioners of judo and wrestling. You should also feel this stretch in your posterior neck and hamstrings.

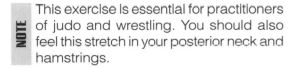 Avoid excessive flexion of the neck.

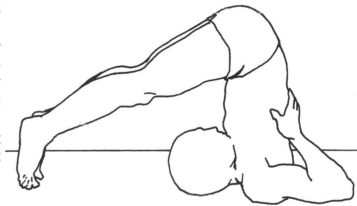

- Lie on your back with your arms by your hips, palms down.
- Inhale, push on the floor with your palms, raise your legs to a vertical position, and support your body with your hands placed on your lower back.
- Exhale, keep your legs straight and together, and lower your feet to the floor.

 This exercise is essential for practitioners of judo and wrestling. You should also feel this stretch in your posterior neck and hamstrings.

Avoid excessive flexion of the neck.

204

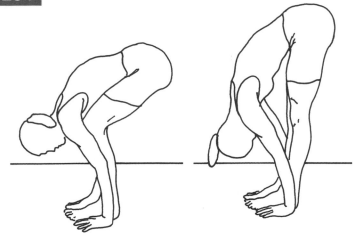

- Squat with your feet and hands resting flat on the floor and your upper torso resting on your thighs.
- Extend your knees until the tension shifts to your hamstrings and then back off.
- Exhale, bend your knees, and return to the starting position.

205

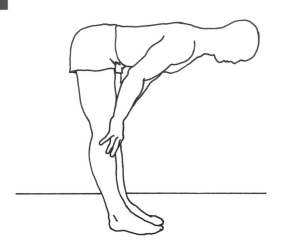

- Stand with your legs straight and your hands by your sides.
- Flex forward at the hips, slide your hands down to your knees, and keep your back flat.
- Exhale and bend your knees or round your upper torso when returning to an upright position.

NOTE You should feel this stretch in both your lower back and hamstrings.

206

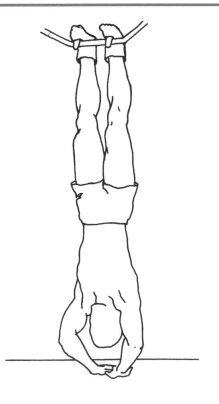

- Wearing inversion boots, hang from a chin-up bar with a forward grip.
- Pull down on the bar, flex your knees, and raise them between your hands so you can hook the boots to the bar. Release the bar and hang from the boots.

⚠️ Don't do inversion stretches if you have glaucoma, hypertension, weakness of blood vessels, or spinal instability. Be sure to receive proper instruction and supervision prior to using any inversion device.

- Kneel on all fours. Straighten your arms, reach forward as far as possible, and lower your chest to the floor.
- Exhale, slightly twist your upper torso, and press your palms and forearms on the floor.

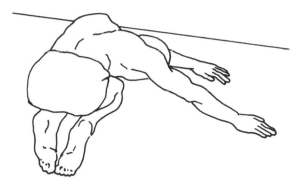

- Sit on a straight-backed chair, turn to your right, and place your hands on the back of the chair.
- Exhale; keeping your feet flat on the floor and your buttocks on the seat, push your right hip forward and press your right elbow into your body.

NOTE You should also feel this stretch in your middle torso.

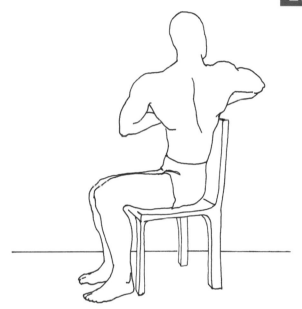

LATERAL TORSO

- Sit on the floor with your legs crossed. Interlock your hands behind your head.
- Exhale and bring your right elbow to your right knee, keeping your left shoulder and elbow back.

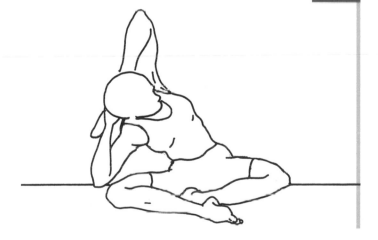

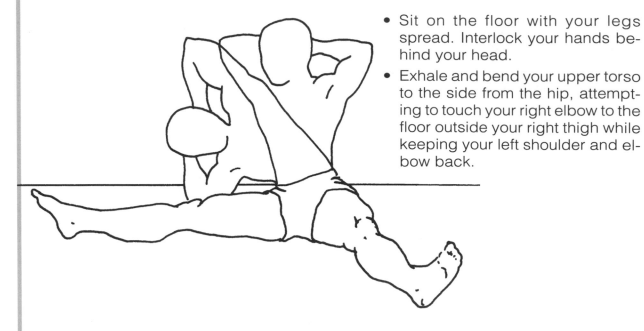

- Sit on the floor with your legs spread. Interlock your hands behind your head.
- Exhale and bend your upper torso to the side from the hip, attempting to touch your right elbow to the floor outside your right thigh while keeping your left shoulder and elbow back.

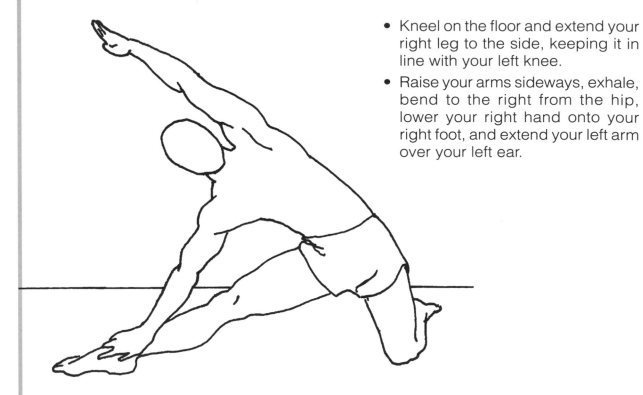

- Kneel on the floor and extend your right leg to the side, keeping it in line with your left knee.
- Raise your arms sideways, exhale, bend to the right from the hip, lower your right hand onto your right foot, and extend your left arm over your left ear.

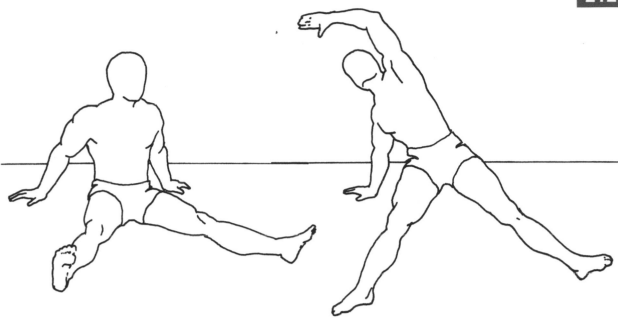

- Sit on the floor with your legs spread, lean backward, and place your hands behind your hips and on the floor for support.
- Inhale, support yourself on your heels, swing your left arm overhead and to the right, and lift your hips off the floor.

- Stand with your feet slightly apart and hands interlocking and overhead.
- Exhale, drop one ear toward your shoulder, and lower your arm sideways.

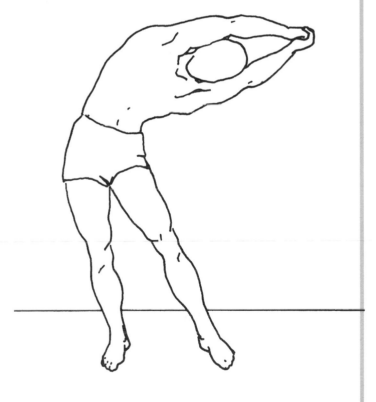

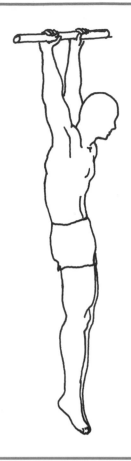

- Hang from a chin-up bar with your arms straight, hands almost touching, and your body in a curved position. Experiment to determine which stretch is more effective: hanging with an overgrip (palms facing forward) or a reverse grip (palms facing backward).

- Exhale, place your chin on your chest, and let your shoulders sink inward.

NOTE You should also feel this stretch in your upper back and shoulders. You can achieve the same effect by hanging from the edge of a baseball dugout.

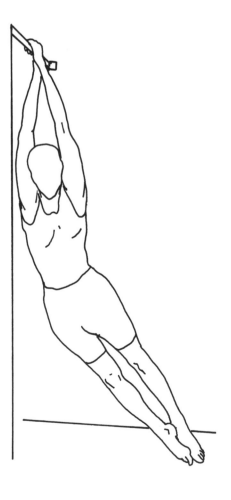

- Hang from a chin-up bar that is lower than head height. Use an overgrip with your hands almost touching.

- Exhale, slide your feet backward, straighten your arms, and hang from the bar with your body arched. Twist your body sideways, keeping your arms behind your ears.

NOTE You should also feel this stretch in your abdomen.

- Hang from a chin-up bar with your arms straight.
- Release one hand at a time and regrasp the bar in an L-grip (the back of the hand facing up and the thumb grasping under the bar).

 NOTE You should also feel this stretch in the brachioradialis.

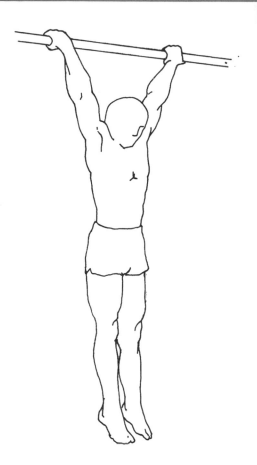

- Lie face down on a table with your hands interlocked behind your head.
- Your partner anchors your pelvis with his hands as you twist your upper torso sideways.

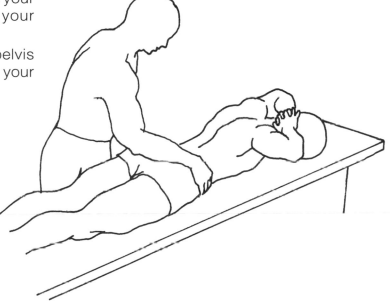

218

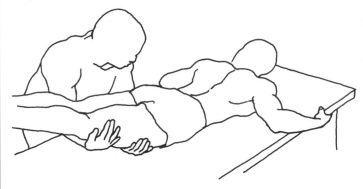

- Lie face down on a table and hold onto the sides for stability.
- Your partner grasps underneath your thighs and lifts your lower torso laterally.

219

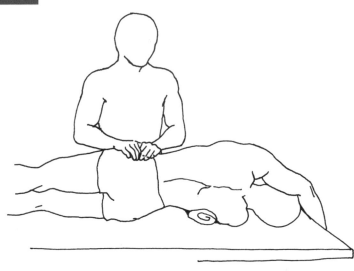

- Lie sideways on a table with your top arm stretched overhead. Use a folded towel to reduce discomfort to your side.
- Your partner anchors your hip as you feel the stretch in the upper lateral torso.

220

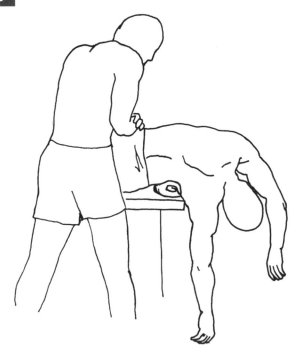

- Lie over the edge of a table with both arms hanging downward. Use a folded towel to reduce discomfort to your side.
- Your partner anchors your hips.

NOTE You should feel the stretch farther down the lateral torso as more of your trunk hangs over the edge.

- Kneel on the floor, extend your right leg to the side, keeping it in line with your left knee, and raise your arm sideways.
- Your partner anchors your hip with one hand and, with the other, grasps your extended arm at about the elbow as he stretches your side.

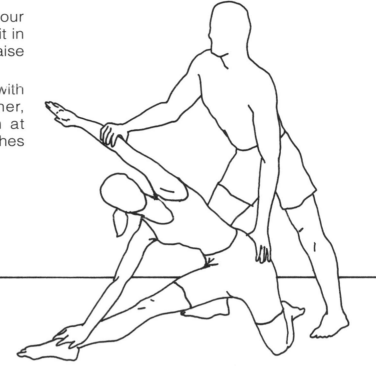

- Stand with your feet slightly apart, one arm by your side and your other arm flexed overhead.
- Your partner anchors your hip with one hand and, with the other, holds your raised arm on or below your elbow.
- Bend your torso to one side with no forward or backward flexing and exhale as your partner pushes your torso farther to one side.

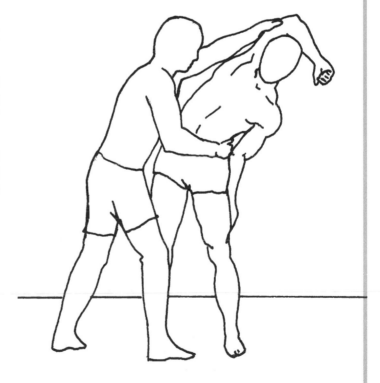

223

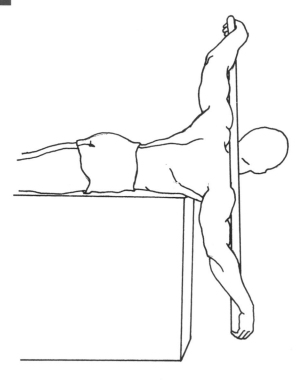

- Lie face down on a table with your upper torso extended over the edge, grasping a stretching stick that rests across your shoulders.
- Exhale as you slowly twist your upper torso as high as possible and return to the starting position.

NOTE This stretch is great for athletes involved in throwing the discus and javelin or swinging a bat, golf club, or racquet.

224

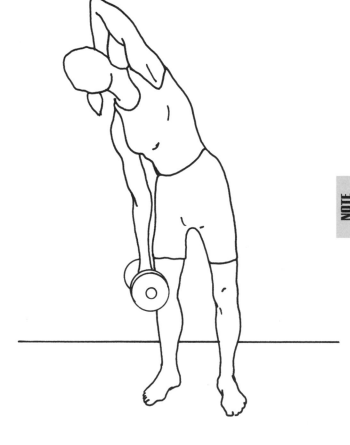

- Stand with your feet parallel and shoulder-width apart, one arm flexed behind your head and your other hand holding a lightweight dumbbell at your side.
- Exhale, maintain your body in a lateral plane, and slowly bend sideways as far as possible.

NOTE You can improvise by using any type of weight (discus, shot put, or a bag containing baseball bats, bowling balls, or golf clubs).

- Stand with your feet parallel and shoulder-width apart and your knees slightly flexed, a lightweight barbell resting across your shoulders.

- Exhale and turn your trunk as far as possible to one side.

⚠️ Turn slowly to reduce momentum that may exceed the absorbing capacity of the tissues being stretched.

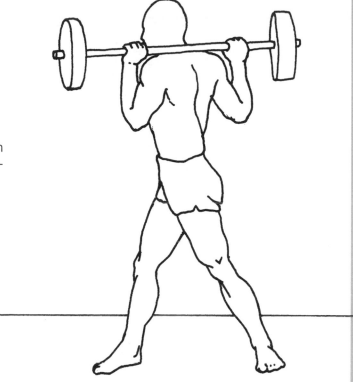

UPPER BACK

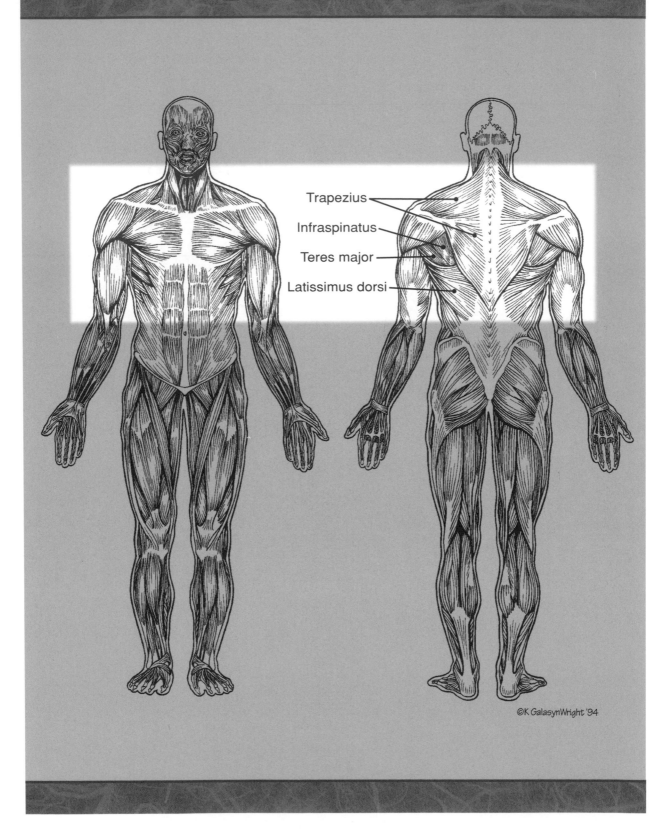

Trapezius

Infraspinatus

Teres major

Latissimus dorsi

©K GalasynWright '94

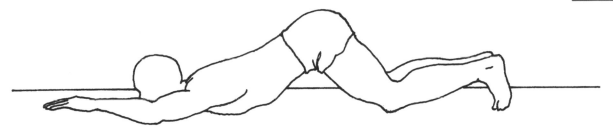

- Kneel on all fours, extend your arms forward, and lower your chest to the floor.
- Exhale, extend your shoulders, and press on the floor with your arms to arch your back.

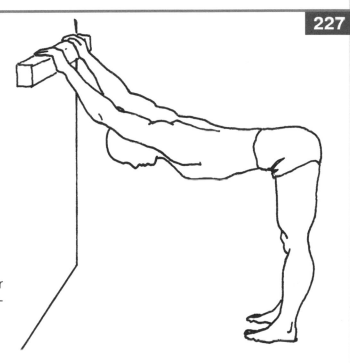

- Stand with your feet together, about three feet (one meter) from a supporting surface approximately hip to shoulder height, and your arms overhead.
- Keeping your arms and legs straight, flex at the hips, flatten your back, and grasp the supporting surface with both hands.
- Exhale and press down on the supporting surface to arch your back.

NOTE You can also stretch your lower back or hamstrings by rotating your pelvis upward.

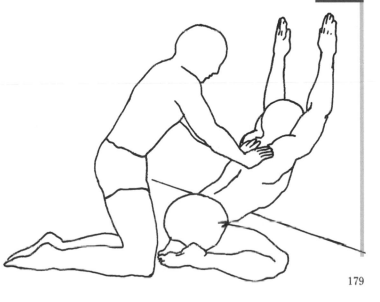

- Sit with knees spread, facing a wall an arm's length away.
- Raise your arms with your elbows straight, lean forward, and place your palms against the wall shoulder-width apart with your fingers pointing upward.
- Exhale, press against the wall, open your chest, and arch your back.
- Your partner places his hands on the upper portion of your shoulder blades and gently pushes down and away from your head.

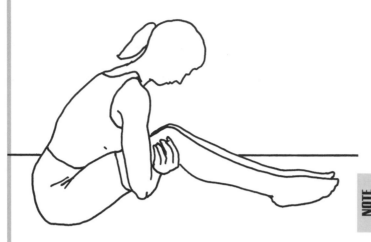

- Sit on the floor with knees slightly flexed, upper torso resting on your thighs, elbows under your knees, and your hands grasping your thighs.
- Exhale, lean forward, and pull back on your thighs while keeping your feet on the floor.

NOTE You should also feel this stretch between the shoulder blades (rhomboids). Round your back to intensify the stretch.

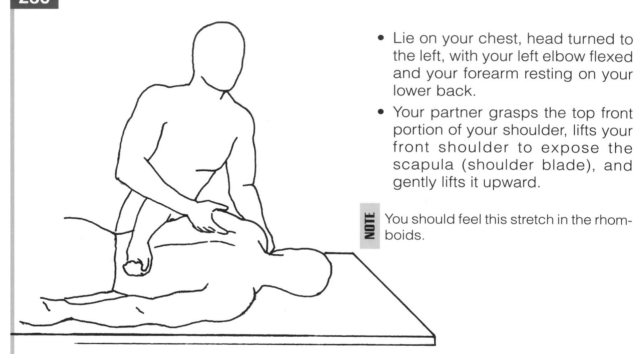

- Lie on your chest, head turned to the left, with your left elbow flexed and your forearm resting on your lower back.
- Your partner grasps the top front portion of your shoulder, lifts your front shoulder to expose the scapula (shoulder blade), and gently lifts it upward.

NOTE You should feel this stretch in the rhomboids.

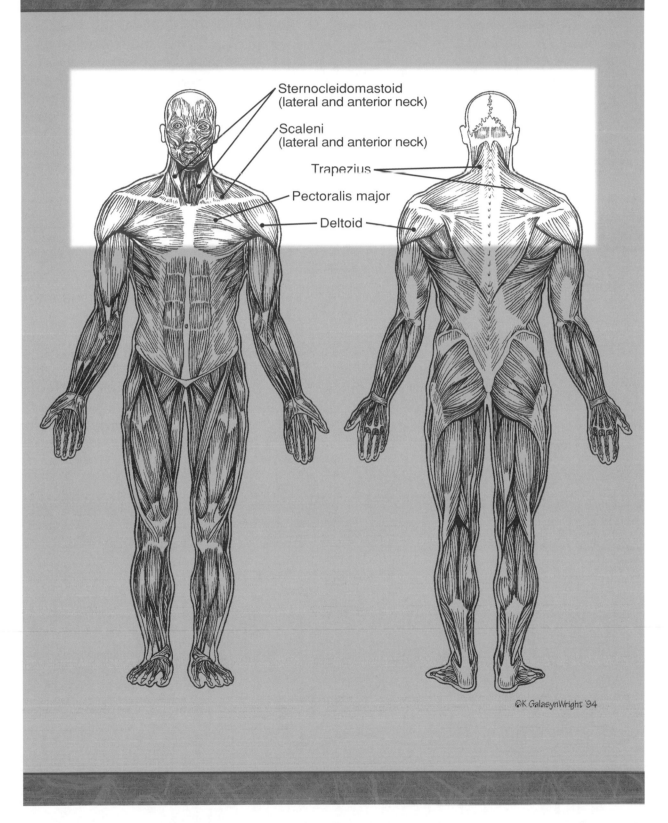

Sternocleidomastoid
(lateral and anterior neck)

Scaleni
(lateral and anterior neck)

Trapezius

Pectoralis major

Deltoid

©K GalasynWright '94

231

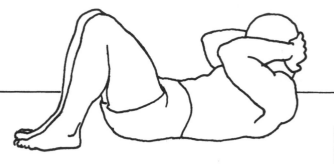

- Lie on the floor on your back with both knees flexed.
- Interlock your hands behind your head near the crown.
- Exhale and pull your head onto your chest while keeping your shoulder blades flat on the floor.

 The stretch will be dissipated if your shoulder blades lift off the floor.

232

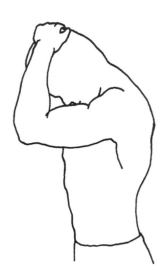

- Stand or sit and interlock your hands behind your head near the crown.
- Exhale, pull your head forward, and allow your chin to rest on your chest. Keep your shoulders depressed during the stretch.

 The stretch will be dissipated if your shoulders do not remain depressed.

233

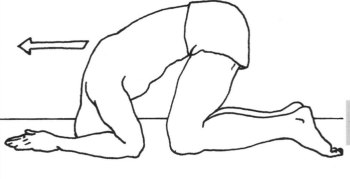

- Kneel on all fours, flex your arms, and place the crown of your head on the floor.
- Exhale, roll your head forward, and bring your chin to your chest.

 This is an essential exercise for those involved in judo and wrestling.

- Lie on your back with your hands by your hips, palms down.
- Exhale, push on the floor with your palms, raise your legs and buttocks off the floor, and extend your legs vertically.
- Bend your elbows and place your hands on your lower back for support.

NOTE This is an essential exercise for those involved in judo and wrestling.

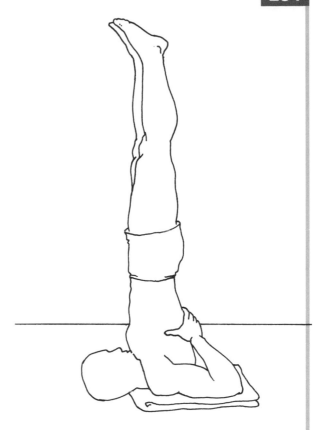

- Lie on your back with your arms by your hips, palms down.
- Exhale, push on the floor with your palms, raise your legs and buttocks off the floor, and extend your legs vertically.
- Bend your elbows and place your hands on your lower back for support.
- Exhale, keep your legs spread, and lower your feet to the floor.

NOTE You should also feel this stretch in your lower back and hamstrings. This is an essential exercise for those involved in judo and wrestling.

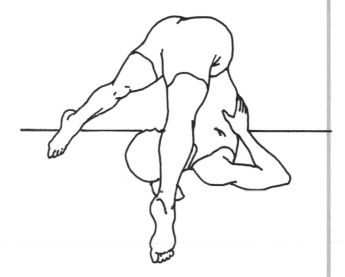

236

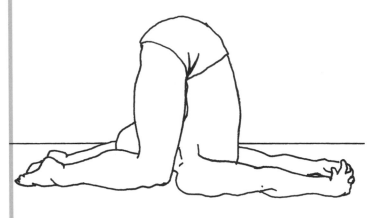

- Lie on your back with your arms by your hips. With your palms pushing down, raise your legs and buttocks off the floor and rest your knees on your forehead.

- Bend your elbows and place your hands on your lower back for support.

- Bring your chin to your chest and flex your knees to the floor on both sides of your ears.

- Exhale, lower your arms to the floor, and interlock your hands.

NOTE This is an essential exercise for those involved in judo and wrestling.

⚠ This exercise may be too advanced or dangerous for even some elite athletes.

237

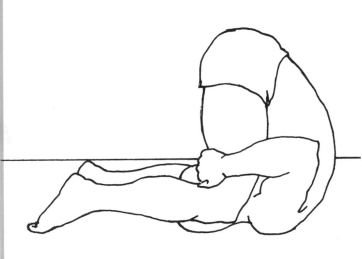

- Lie on your back with your arms by your hips. With your palms pushing down, raise your legs and buttocks off the floor and rest your knees on your forehead.

- Bend your elbows and place your hands on your lower back for support.

- Bring your chin to your chest and flex your knees to the floor on both sides of your ears.

- Exhale, put your hands behind your knees, and pull your thighs to your chest while resting your knees and shins on the floor.

NOTE This is an essential exercise for those involved in judo and wrestling.

- Lie on your back with your arms by your hips. With your palms pushing down, raise your legs and buttocks off the floor and rest your knees on your forehead.
- Bend your elbows and place your hands on your lower back for support.
- Bring your chin to your chest, flex your knees to the left side of your head, and rest your knees and shins on the floor.

NOTE This is an essential exercise for those involved in judo and wrestling.

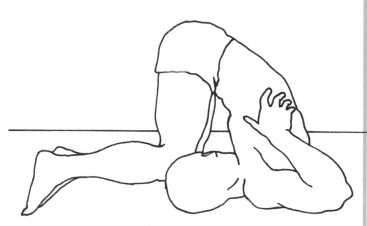

- Stand with your feet together holding a pair of lightweight dumbbells by your hips.
- Exhale and let your shoulders sink as low as possible. Draw your chin in to rest on your chest.

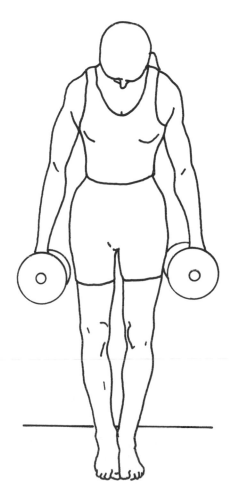

240

- Stand with your feet together holding a light barbell in front of your body with your hands touching.
- Exhale and let your shoulders sink as low as possible. Draw your chin in to rest on your chest.

NOTE You can also use any weighted sports equipment instead of a barbell, such as a discus, shot put, or a bag containing baseball bats, bowling balls, or golf clubs.

241

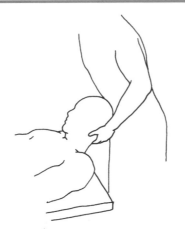

- Lie on your back on the floor or on a table with your head hanging over the edge.
- Your partner holds the back of your head with both hands.
- Exhale as your partner gently lifts your head and brings it to your chest.

LATERAL NECK

242

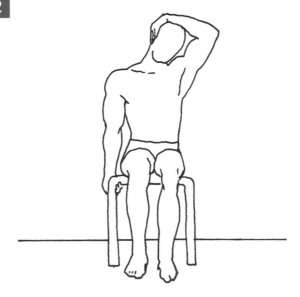

- Sit on a chair with your right hand grasping the lowest part of the chair frame to stabilize your right shoulder.
- Place your left hand on the upper right side of your head.
- Exhale and pull the left side of your head onto your left shoulder.

NOTE The stretch will be dissipated upon release of the chair.

- Sit or stand with your left arm flexed behind your back.
- Grasp the elbow from behind with the opposite hand and pull it across the midline of your back to keep your left shoulder stabilized.
- Exhale and lower your right ear to your right shoulder.

 NOTE The stretch will be dissipated upon release of the anchored shoulder.

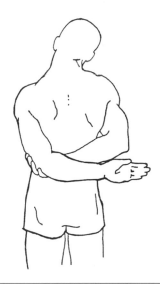

- Stand with your feet together, holding a lightweight dumbbell in your right hand.
- Exhale and let your right shoulder sink as low as possible as you place your left hand on the upper right side of your head.
- Exhale and pull the left side of your head onto your left shoulder.

 NOTE Keep your left shoulder fixed.

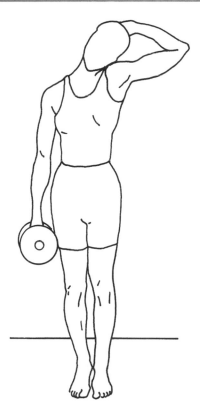

ANTERIOR NECK

- Lie on your back on a table with your head hanging over the edge.
- Hold the stretch and relax.

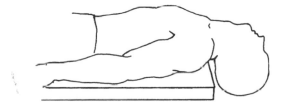

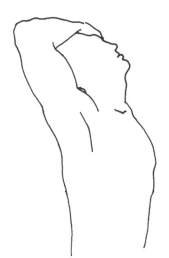

- Sit or stand and carefully lean your head back.
- Place your hands on your forehead, exhale, and gently pull your head backward.

NOTE This exercise is important for those involved in judo or wrestling.

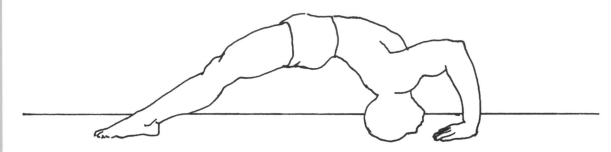

- Lie on your back with your heels close to your hips, the palms of your hands on the floor under your shoulders, and your fingers pointing toward your feet.
- Inhale, raise your trunk, and rest your forehead on the floor.
- Exhale and roll your head backward.

NOTE This this is an essential exercise for those involved in judo and wrestling.

PECTORALS

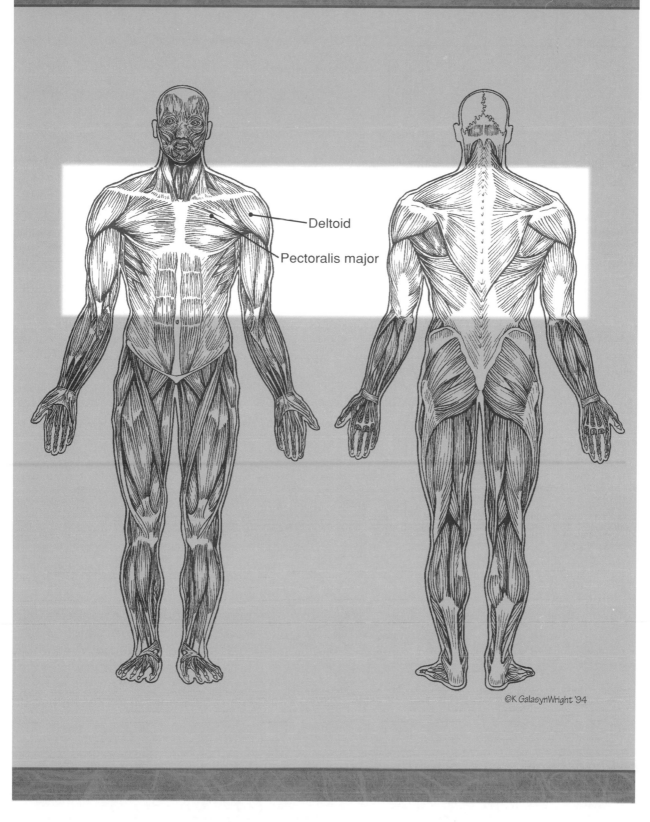

Deltoid

Pectoralis major

©K GalasynWright '94

248

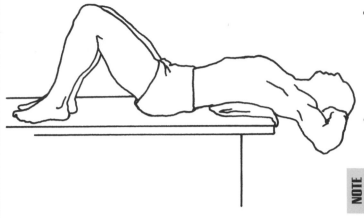

- Lie on a table with a folded blanket under your upper back, your legs flexed, your upper torso hanging over the edge, and your hands interlocked behind your head.

- Exhale and lower your head and shoulders toward the floor.

NOTE Keep your neck extended and your elbows abducted. Also, if necessary, a partner can anchor your feet.

249

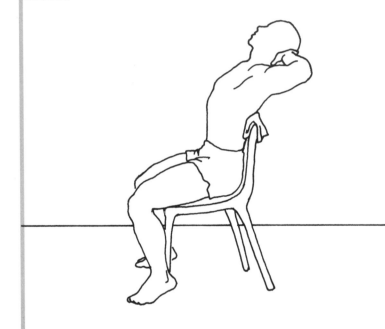

- Sit on a chair with your hands interlocked behind your head and the top of the chair at midchest level.

- Inhale, lean your upper torso backward, and pull your arms backward.

250

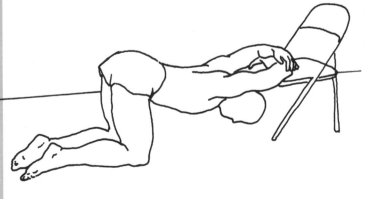

- Kneel on the floor facing a barre or chair.

- Interlock your forearms above your head and bend forward to rest them on top of the barre or chair, with your head dropping beneath the surface. Exhale and let your head and chest sink to the floor.

- Stand facing a corner or open doorway.
- Raise your elbows in a reverse *T* (elbows below your shoulders) to stretch the collarbone section of the pectoral muscles bilaterally.
- Exhale and lean your entire body forward.

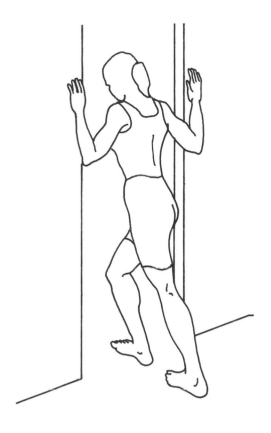

- Stand facing a corner or open doorway.
- Raise your elbows to shoulder height at your sides, bend your elbows so that your forearms point straight up, and place your palms against the walls or door frame to stretch the sternal section of the pectoral muscles on both sides. This position will form the letter *T*.
- Exhale and lean your entire body forward.

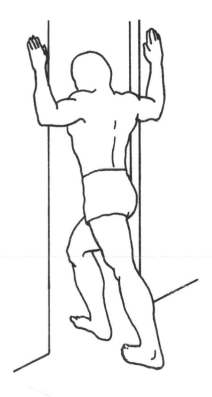

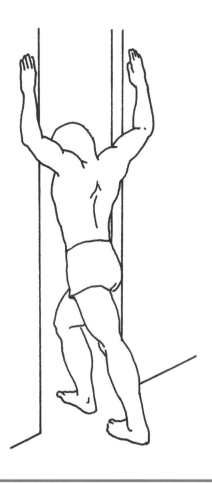

- Stand facing a corner or open doorway.
- Raise your elbows above shoulder height at your sides to form the letter *V*, slightly flex your elbows, and place your palms against the walls or door frame to stretch the rib section of the pectoral muscles on both sides.
- Exhale and lean your entire body forward.

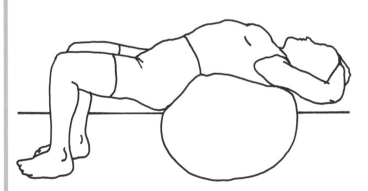

- Sit on the floor with a large Swiss ball against your lower back and your hands interlocked behind your head, elbows facing forward.
- Inhale, extend your thighs, raise your buttocks off the floor, roll the ball, and achieve a neutral position. The ball should be under your shoulder blades (scapula), with your lumbar spine flat, your knees flexed at 90 degrees, and your elbows abducted.

 NOTE You should feel the stretch in the upper chest and thoracic area.

- Sit with both arms flexed and your hands interlocked behind your head.
- Your partner grasps both elbows and pulls them backward toward each other.

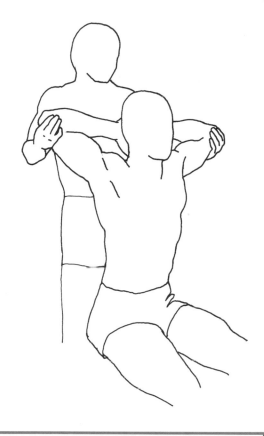

- Lie on a bench with your legs flexed and your feet resting on its surface.
- Hold two lightweight dumbbells directly over your chest with your arms straight and knuckles facing out.
- Keeping your arms slightly flexed, lower the dumbbells sideways, moving your elbows until they are level with your shoulders. Exhale and return to the starting position, bringing the dumbbells back up in an arc.

 NOTE You can also execute these "flys" with straight arms.

 This exercise can apply extreme tension to the elbow and shoulder joints.

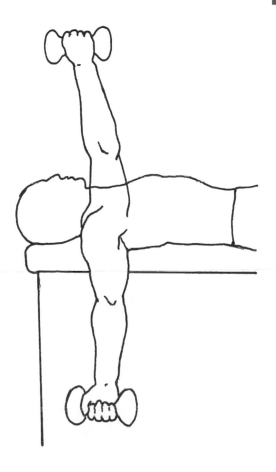

SHOULDERS

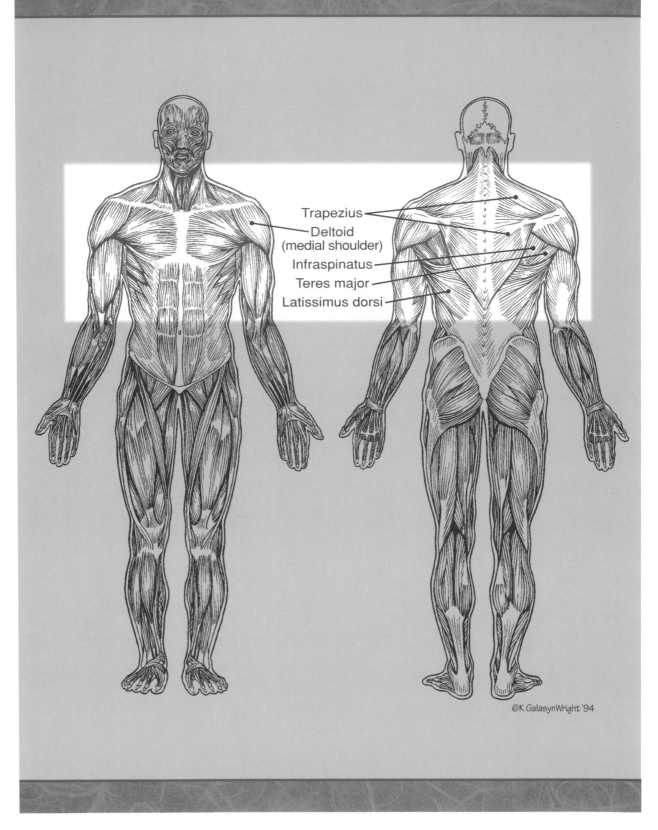

Trapezius
Deltoid
(medial shoulder)
Infraspinatus
Teres major
Latissimus dorsi

©K GalasynWright '94

257

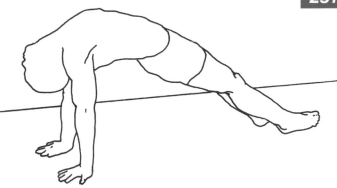

- Sit on the floor with your hands about one foot (30 centimeters) behind your hips, your fingers pointing away from your body, and your legs extended forward.
- Inhale, lift your buttocks, raise your trunk off the floor, and open your chest as wide as possible.

258

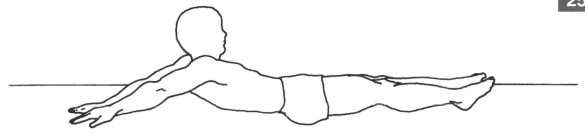

- Sit on the floor with your hands about one foot (30 centimeters) behind your hips, your fingers pointing away from your body, palms down, and your legs extended forward.
- Exhale, slide your buttocks forward, and lean backward as far as possible.

259

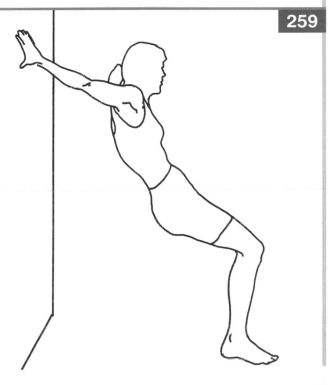

- Stand with your hands behind your back, resting on a wall at about shoulder height, and your fingers pointing upward.
- Exhale, flex your legs, and lower your shoulders.

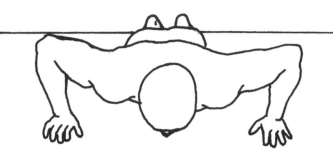

260

- Assume a push-up position with your arms as wide as possible.
- Exhale and lower your chest almost to the floor before returning to the starting position.

NOTE This stretch requires adequate strength to support oneself.

261

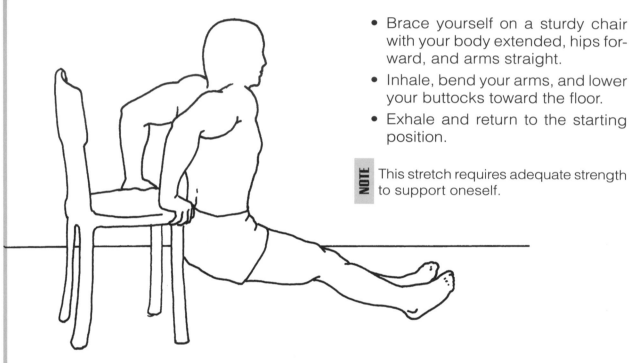

- Brace yourself on a sturdy chair with your body extended, hips forward, and arms straight.
- Inhale, bend your arms, and lower your buttocks toward the floor.
- Exhale and return to the starting position.

NOTE This stretch requires adequate strength to support oneself.

- Hang from a pair of still rings, inhale, and raise your body to an inverted hang.
- Exhale and lower your legs to the floor (skin the cat). Sink as low as possible in the shoulders.

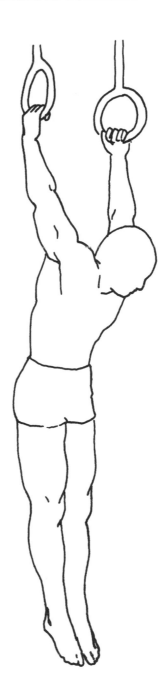

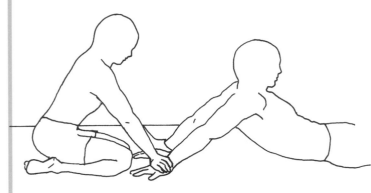

263

- Sit on the floor with your hands about 12 inches (30 centimeters) behind your hips, your fingers pointing away from your body, palms down, and your legs extended forward.
- Your partner kneels directly behind you and holds both wrists.
- Exhale as your partner gently pulls your arms backward and downward.

NOTE Be sure to communicate with your partner. It is not necessary for the wrists to touch each other.

⚠️ Stretching to the point where the elbows cross behind the back has been criticized for increasing the likelihood of anterior dislocation in swimmers.

264

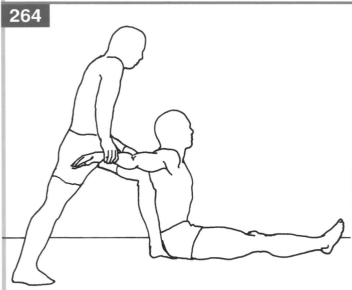

- Sit or kneel on the floor with your arms raised horizontally behind your back.
- Your partner holds both wrists and gently pulls your arms backward in a horizontal plane.

NOTE It is not necessary for the wrists to contact each other.

⚠️ Stretching to the point where the elbows cross behind the back has been criticized for increasing the likelihood of anterior dislocation in swimmers.

265

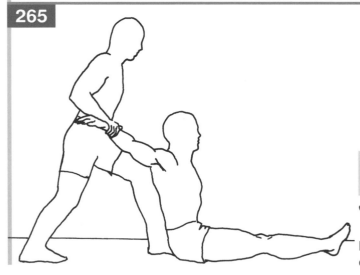

- Sit or kneel on the floor with your arms raised above horizontal behind your back.
- Exhale as your partner gently pulls your arms backward and upward.

NOTE It is not necessary for the wrists to contact each other.

⚠️ Stretching to the point where the elbows cross behind the back has been criticized for increasing the likelihood of anterior dislocation in swimmers.

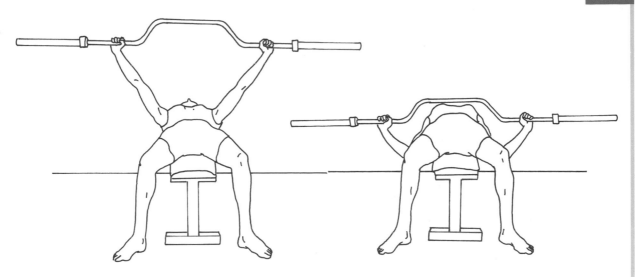

- Lie on a bench with your legs resting on the floor. Hold an unweighted cambered Olympic bar with your arms straight.
- Inhale and lower the bar until it almost contacts your anterior neck, then exhale and return the bar to its starting position.

 NOTE The cambered Olympic bar is a bar specially designed for weight lifting.

- Stand with your legs together. Grasp a pole or towel in front of your hips with a wide overgrip (palms facing down).
- Inhale and raise your arms overhead, keeping them straight and symmetrical, with no twisting to the side as they rotate in the shoulder joint and end up behind your hips.
- Inhale, then reverse the direction.

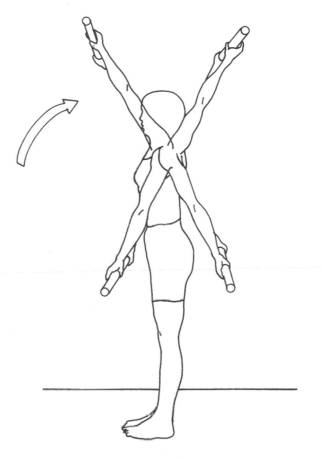

MEDIAL SHOULDER (DELTOIDS)

268

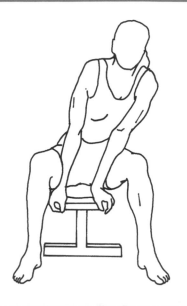

- Sit on a bench with both arms straight, hands flat on the bench surface, and shoulders externally rotated.
- Exhale, weight your arms by lowering your body, and lean toward one side and then the other.

LATERAL SHOULDER

269

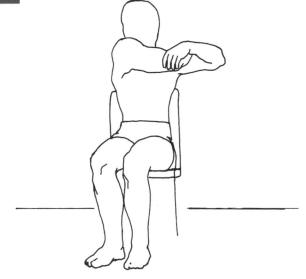

- Sit or stand with one arm raised to shoulder height; flex the arm across to the other shoulder.
- Grasp your raised elbow with the opposite hand, exhale, and pull your elbow backward.

NOTE Experiment with flexing and extending the arm of the stretched shoulder to find the most effective stretch.

270

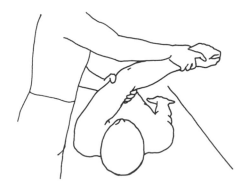

- Lie on your back on a table with one arm raised vertically.
- Your partner grasps your elbow with one hand and your wrist with the other and pushes your extended arm across your chest.

271

- Sit with your side next to a table and rest your forearm along the table edge with your elbow flexed.
- Exhale, bend forward from the hips, and lower your head and shoulder to table level.

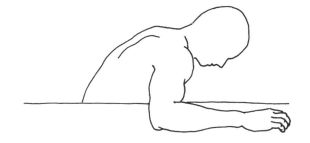

272

- Stand facing the edge of a door frame. Flex your elbow and place your hand on the frame.
- Exhale and turn away from your fixed arm as it remains against your side.

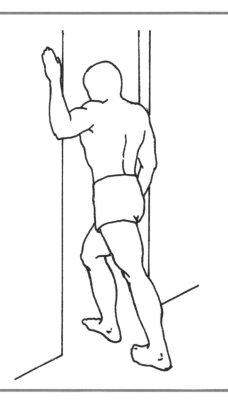

273

- Lie on your back on a table and flex your arm with your elbow resting over the edge.
- Your partner anchors your elbow with one hand and gently pushes downward on your wrist with the other.

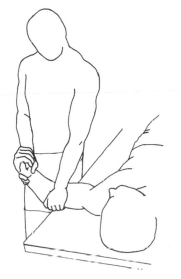

274

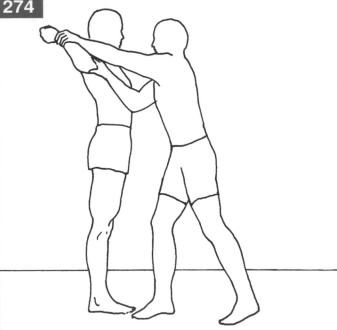

- Stand with your right arm raised to shoulder height and flexed at a right angle.
- Your partner pushes your right wrist backward and downward with his left hand while supporting your right elbow with his right hand.

275

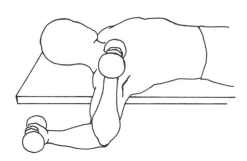

- Lie on a bench or table with your arm resting over the edge and your elbow flexed at a 90-degree angle while holding a lightweight dumbbell.
- Inhale and lower the weight until parallel with your head, then exhale and return to the starting position.

⚠️ Do not do this stretch if you have recently suffered an anterior shoulder dislocation. The stretch should be done only after the injury has healed, and then with a partner providing support under the wrist.

SHOULDER EXTERNAL ROTATORS (POSTERIOR)

276

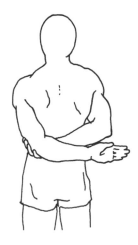

- Sit or stand with one arm flexed behind your back and grasp the elbow from behind with your opposite hand.
- Exhale and pull your elbow across the midline of your back. Grasp your wrist if you are unable to reach your elbow.

- Sit or stand, flex your right arm, and raise your elbow to chest height.
- Flex and raise your left arm so its elbow can support your right elbow and intertwine your forearms so your left hand grasps your right wrist.
- Exhale and pull your wrist outward and downward.

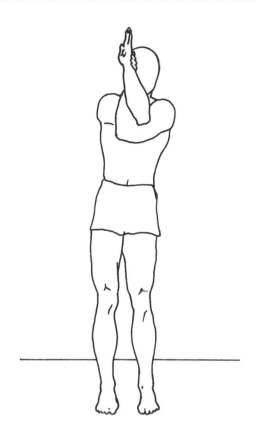

- Sit on a chair with a firm back and place one arm behind the back at about waist level.
- Exhale and turn your head and rotate your trunk toward the stretched side.

NOTE To increase this stretch, gently push your elbow against the back of the chair. After each successive contraction, rotate your trunk a bit farther in the direction of the arm being stretched.

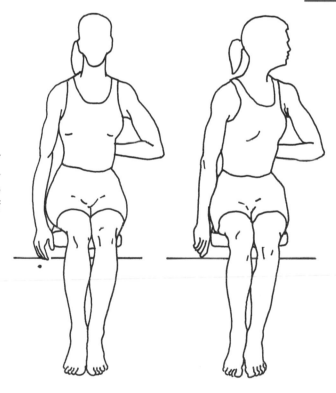

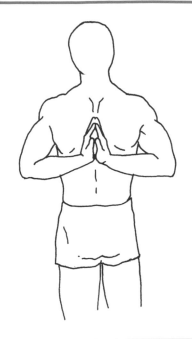

- Sit or stand and place your palms together behind your back with your fingers pointing downward.
- Inhale, rotate your wrists so your fingers are pointing toward your head, and draw your elbows back.

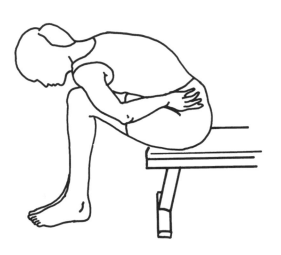

- Sit on a chair with your legs together and your feet flat on the floor. Place both hands on your hips with the thumbs facing forward.
- Bend forward from the hips and rest the anterior part of your shoulders on your knees.
- Exhale and let your elbows move forward and attempt to touch each other.

 NOTE Intensify this stretch by stretching one shoulder and having the opposite hand grasp and pull down on the elbow.

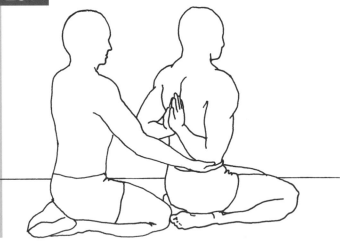

- Sit or kneel with your palms together behind your back and your fingers pointing downward.
- Inhale; rotate your wrists so your fingers are pointing toward your head as your partner pulls both elbows backward.

- Stand with one arm behind your back, the thumb pointing up, reaching your hand as close as possible to the opposite shoulder.
- With one hand anchored against your scapula and the other hand grasping your wrist, your partner gently pulls your hand away from your back.

NOTE Be sure to communicate with your partner.

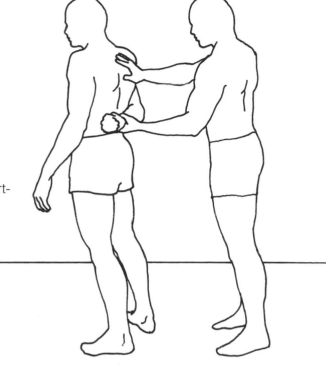

- Lie on your back on a table and flex your arm and rest your elbow over the edge.
- Your partner anchors your elbow with one hand and grasps your wrist with the other.
- Exhale as your partner gently pushes your hand forward and downward toward your feet.

NOTE Communicate with your partner and use great care.

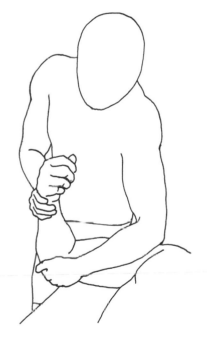

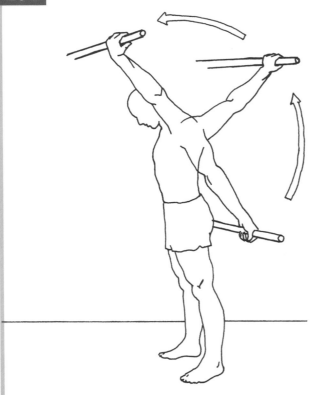

- Stand with your feet spread and grasp a pole or towel with both hands behind your hips in a wide reverse grip (your palms facing forward and thumbs on the outside).

- Straighten and raise your arms overhead, keeping both symmetrical, without twisting to the side as your arms rotate forward in the shoulder joint and end in an L-grip (the palms of the hands facing up and the thumbs under the pole).

- Inhale, then reverse the direction.

NOTE This is an important stretch for gymnasts who work on the horizontal bar.

SHOULDER EXTENSORS

285

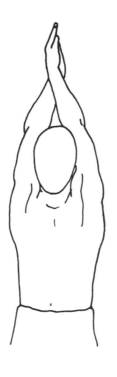

- Sitting or standing, cross one wrist over the other and interlock your hands.

- Inhale, then straighten and extend your arms behind your head. Your elbows should be behind your ears.

- Hang from a chin-up bar with your arms straight, hands in an overgrip (palms facing forward) and touching, and your body in a curved position.
- Exhale, keep your arms straight, flex at the hips, and raise your knees; place your chin on your chest, position your elbows behind your head, and let your shoulders sink inward.

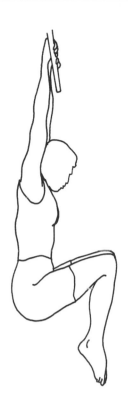

 NOTE Keep your hands together, your body straight, and your head behind your arms for the most effective stretch. This stretch can be enhanced by developing a small swing.

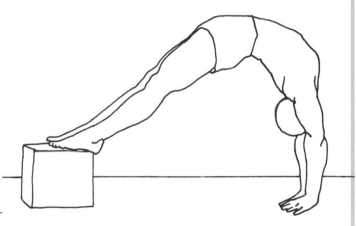

- Lie on your back with your feet resting on a block or sturdy bench, your hands on the floor by your neck (under the shoulders), and your fingers pointing toward your feet.
- Inhale and raise your torso off the floor into a full bridge.
- Exhale and extend your shoulders past your wrists (vertical).

NOTE You should feel this stretch in the abdomen, shoulders, and upper thigh.

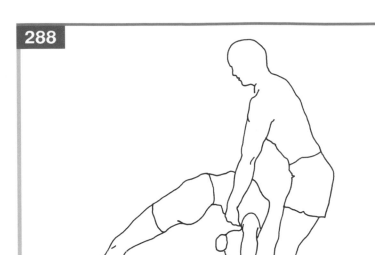

- Lie on your back, with your heels close to your hips. Grasp the ankles of your partner, who stands straddling your head.
- Inhale, extend your arms and legs, and raise your body into a full bridge.
- Your partner interlocks his hands beneath your shoulders and lifts you upward and forward.

NOTE You should feel this stretch in the abdomen, shoulders, and upper thigh.

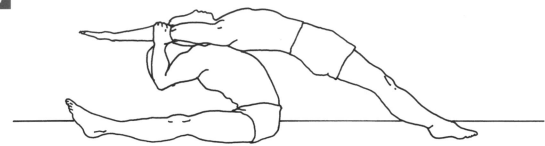

- Sit upright on the floor with your legs straight and your arms parallel and overhead.
- Your partner sits on the floor, back-to-back with you in the same position, grasping your arms above the elbows.
- Exhale as you allow your partner to lean forward, pull, and lift your torso off the floor.

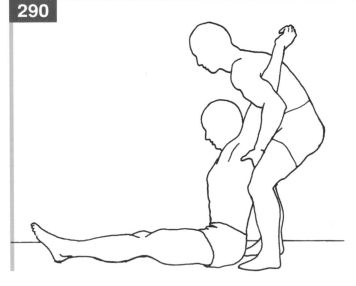

- Sit on the floor with your arms parallel and overhead.
- Your partner braces his knees against your spine, hooks your elbows in his armpits, and places his hands on your upper shoulder blades.
- Exhale as your partner pushes your shoulder blades forward and pulls your arms backward.

NOTE You should feel this stretch in the chest, shoulders, and upper back.

- Kneel on the floor with your arms parallel, overhead, and touching your ears.
- Your partner straddles your legs from behind.
- Grasp your partner around the neck and interlock your hands as the partner lifts up and leans backward.

 NOTE You should feel this stretch in the chest, shoulders, upper back, and abdomen.

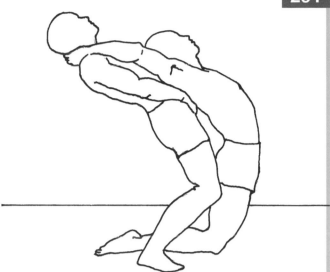

- Stand with your feet together and your arms parallel, overhead, and touching your ears.
- Your partner stands back-to-back with you. With knees flexed and buttocks beneath yours, he reaches upward and grasps your arms between the elbows and shoulders.
- Exhale as your partner gently leans forward, slightly straightens his legs, and lifts you off the floor.

 NOTE You should feel this stretch in the chest, shoulders, upper back, and abdomen.

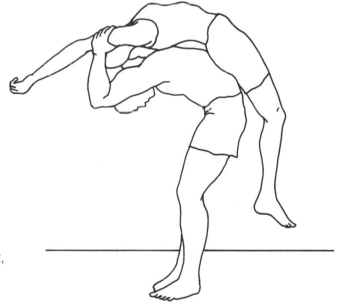

- Lie on your back on a bench. Hold a lightweight dumbbell on your lower chest with both hands.
- Exhale and raise the dumbbell off your chest.
- Inhale, straighten your arms, and lower the dumbbell over your head as close to the floor as possible.
- Exhale and return to the starting point.

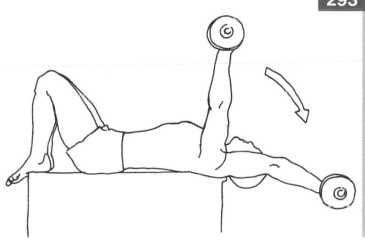

ARMS AND WRISTS

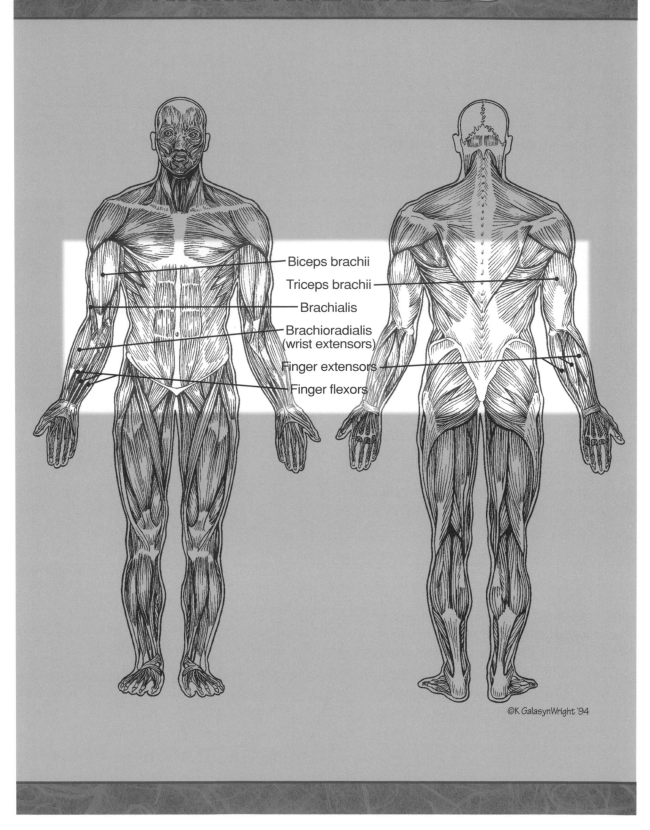

Biceps brachii

Triceps brachii

Brachialis

Brachioradialis
(wrist extensors)

Finger extensors

Finger flexors

©K GalasynWright '94

294

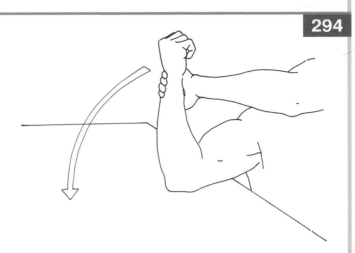

- Sit with one arm flexed to 90 degrees and your elbow resting on a table; grasp your wrist with the opposite hand.
- Exhale and contract the biceps as you stretch them with your other hand (eccentric contraction).
- When your arm is fully extended, hold the stretch and relax.

295

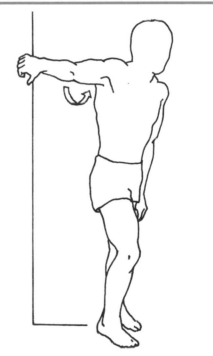

- Stand with your back to a door frame.
- Rest one hand against the door frame with your arm internally rotated at the shoulder, your forearm extended, and your hand pronated with your thumb pointing down. Exhale and attempt to roll your biceps so they face upward.

296

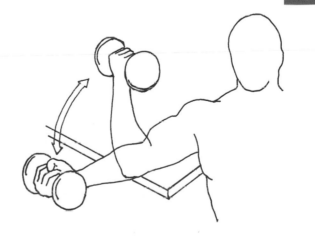

- Sit or stand by a table holding a light-weight dumbbell with your forearm resting on the table surface and your elbow flexed to 90 degrees.
- Inhale and extend your elbow while contracting your biceps (eccentric contraction).
- Exhale and return the weight to the starting position.

NOTE This stretch may result in muscle soreness!

297

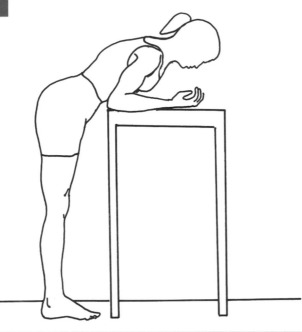

- Stand with your forearms resting on a table, palms facing up.
- Exhale, bend forward, and bring your shoulders to your wrist.

298

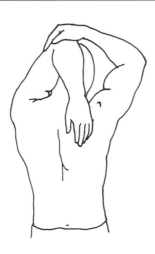

- Sit or stand with one arm flexed, raised overhead next to your ear, and your hand resting on your shoulder blade.
- Grasp your elbow with the other hand, exhale, and pull your elbow behind your head.

 NOTE This stretch is most effective when the raised elbow is against a wall.

299

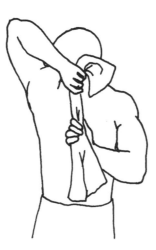

- Sit or stand with one arm behind your lower back and as far up on your back as possible.
- Lift your other arm overhead while holding a folded blanket or towel and flex your elbow.
- Grasp the blanket or towel with your lower hand and inhale as you pull your hands toward each other.

 NOTE This stretch is most effective when the raised elbow is against a wall.

- Sit or stand with one arm behind your back and as far up on your back as possible.
- Lift your other arm overhead, flex your elbow, and interlock your fingers.

NOTE This stretch is most effective when the raised elbow is against a wall.

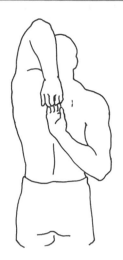

- Sit on the floor with your legs spread; raise your right arm and flex it behind your head.
- Flex your left arm across your chest and inhale as your partner pulls down on your raised elbow and across on your opposite elbow.

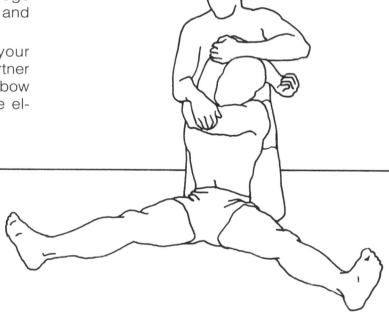

- Sit or stand with one arm flexed and raised overhead next to your ear and your hand resting on your shoulder blade.
- Your partner grasps your wrist with one hand and holds your elbow with the other.
- Exhale as your partner gently raises your elbow and pulls your wrist downward.

NOTE Be sure to communicate with your partner and use great care.

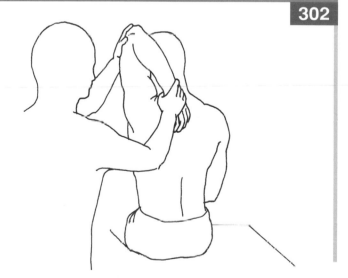

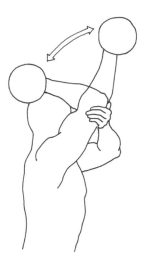

303

- Sit and hold a lightweight dumbbell overhead with one hand as the other hand supports your elbow.
- Inhale as you lower the dumbbell behind your head. Exhale as you return to the starting position.

WRIST EXTENSORS (BRACHIORADIALIS)

304

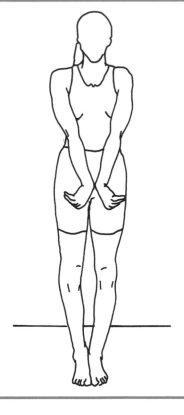

- Stand with your arms straight and your palms facing each other.
- Exhale and rotate your hands and wrists inward.

NOTE You may wish to rotate your hands and wrists rhythmically.

305

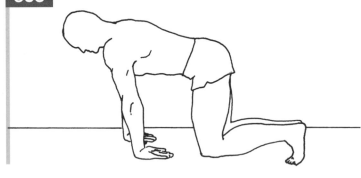

- Kneel on all fours, flex your wrists, and place the tops of your hands against the floor, fingers pointing toward your knees.
- Exhale and lean against the floor.

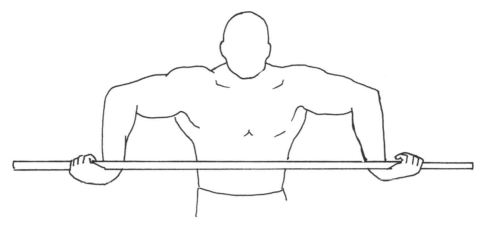

- Hold a pole above your head with your hands in an L-grip (the back of the hand facing up and the thumbs grasping under the pole).
- Exhale and lower the pole in front of your body to your waist while flexing your elbows.

 Modify this stretch by using a bat, racquet, or golf club of appropriate length.

- Hang from a chin-up bar with your arms straight.
- Release one hand and regrasp the bar in an L-grip.

 You should feel this stretch in the lats as well as the brachioradialis. If the stretch is too uncomfortable, stand on a chair to reduce the intensity.

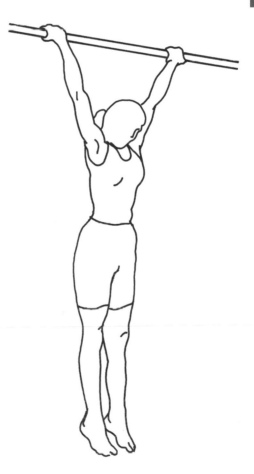

308

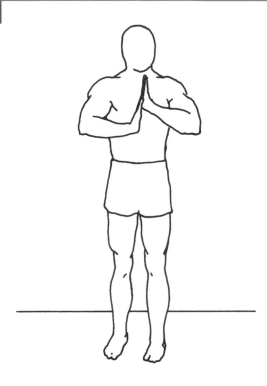

- Sit or stand on the floor with your wrists bent backward.
- Place the heel of one hand against the upper portion of the fingers of your other hand, and press the heel of your hand against your fingers.

309

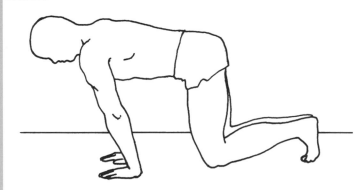

- Kneel on all fours, flex your wrists, and place your palms against the floor, fingers pointed away from your body.
- Exhale and lean forward.

310

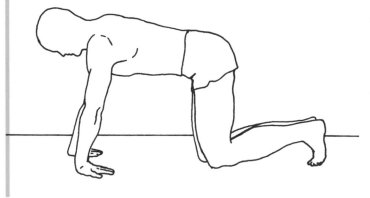

- Kneel on all fours, flex your wrists, and place your palms against the floor with the fingers pointing toward your body.
- Exhale and lean backward.

- Kneel on all fours, flex your wrists, and place your palms against the floor with the heel of each hand touching the other.
- Exhale and lean forward and backward.

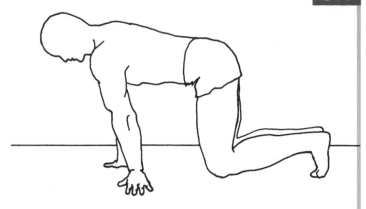

REFERENCES

Adler, S.S., D. Beckers, and M. Buck. 1993. *PNF in practice: An illustrated guide.* New York: Springer-Verlag.

Akeson, W.H., D. Amiel, and S. Woo. 1980. Immobility effects on synovial joints: The pathomechanics of joint contracture. *Biorheology* 17(1): 95-110.

Alter, M.J. 1996. *Science of flexibility.* Champaign, IL: Human Kinetics.

Aten, D.W., and K.T. Knight. 1978. Therapeutic exercise in athletic training: Principles and overview. *Athletic Training* 13(3): 123-126.

Bandy, W.D., and J.M. Irion. 1994. The effect of time on static stretch on the flexibility of the hamstring muscles. *Physical Therapy* 74(9): 845-852.

Brooks, G.A., and T.D. Fahey. 1987. *Fundamentals of human performance.* New York: Macmillan.

Cohen, D.B., M.A. Mont, K.R. Campbell, B.N. Vogelstein, and J.W. Loewy. 1994. Upper extremity physical factors affecting tennis serve velocity. *American Journal of Sports Medicine* 22(6): 746-750.

Cook, E.E., V.L. Gray, E. Savinar-Nogue, and J. Medeiros. 1987. Shoulder antagonistic strength ratios: A comparison between college level baseball pitchers and nonpitchers. *Journal of Orthopaedic and Sports Physical Therapy* 8(9): 451-461.

Cornelius, W.L., R.W. Hagemann, and A.W. Jackson. 1988. A study on placement of stretching within a workout. *Journal of Sports Medicine and Physical Fitness* 28(3): 234-236.

Costill, D.L., E.W. Maglischo, and A.B. Richardson. 1992. *Swimming: Handbook of sport medicine and science.* Oxford: Blackwell.

de Vries, H.A. 1961. Electromyographic observation of the effect of static stretching upon muscular distress. *Research Quarterly* 32(4): 468-479.

———. 1966. Quantitative electromyographic investigation of spasm theory of muscular pain. *American Journal of Physical Medicine* 45(3): 119-134

Goldspink, G. 1968. Sarcomere length during post-natal growth and mammalian muscle fibres. *Journal of Cell Science* 3(4): 539-548.

Halbertsma, J.P.K., A.I. van Bolhuis, and L.N.H. Göeken. 1996. Sport stretching: Effect on passive muscle stiffness of short hamstrings. *Archives of Physical Medicine and Rehabilitation* 77(7): 688-692.

Halbertsma, J.P.K., and L.N.H. Göeken. 1994. Stretching exercises: Effect on passive extensibility and stiffness in short hamstrings of healthy subjects. *Archives of Physical Medicine and Rehabilitation* 75(9): 976-981.

Hardy, L. 1985. Improving active range of hip flexion. *Research Quarterly for Exercise and Sport* 56(2): 111-114.

Harre, D. 1982. *Principles of sports training.* Berlin: Sportverlag.

Huxley, H.E., and J. Hanson. 1954. Changes in cross-striations of muscles during contraction and stretch and their structural interpretation. *Nature* 173(4412): 973-976.

Iashvili, A.V. 1983. Active and passive flexibility in athletes specializing in different sports. *Soviet Sports Review* 18(1): 30-32.

Johns, R.J., and V. Wright. 1962. Relative importance of various tissues in joint stiffness. *Journal of Applied Physiology* 17(5): 824-828.

Karmenov, B. 1990. Knee-joint mobility. *Soviet Sports Review* 25(4): 200-201.

Kurz, T. 1994. *Stretching scientifically: A guide to flexibility training* (3rd ed.). Island Pond, VT: Stadion.

Lubell, A. 1989. Potentially dangerous exercises: Are they harmful to all? *The Physician and Sportsmedicine* 17(1): 187-192.

Magnusson, S.P., E.B. Simonsen, P. Aagaard, P. Dyhre-Poulsen, M.P. McHugh, and M. Kjaer. 1996. Mechanical and physiological responses to stretching with and without preisometric contraction in human skeletal muscle. *Archives of Physical Medicine and Rehabilitation* 77(4): 373-378.

Matveyev, L. 1981. *Fundamentals of sports training.* Moscow: Progress.

McAtee, R.E. 1993. *Facilitated stretching.* Champaign, IL: Human Kinetics.

Merni, F., M. Balboni, S. Bargellini, and G. Menegatti. 1981. Differences in males and females in joint movement range during growth. *Medicine and Sport* 15: 168-175.

Moore, J.C. 1984. The Golgi tendon organ: A review and update. *American Journal of Occupational Therapy* 38(4): 227-236.

Moore, M.A., and R.S. Hutton. 1980. Electromyographic investigation of muscle stretching techniques. *Medicine and Science in Sports and Exercise* 12(5): 322-329.

Moore, M.A., and C.G. Kukulka. 1991. Depression of Hoffman reflexes following voluntary contraction and implications for proprioceptive neuromuscular facilitation therapy. *Physical Therapy* 71(4): 321-333.

Myers, E.R., C.G. Armstrong, and V.C. Mow, 1984, Swelling, pressure, and collagen tension. In *Connective tissue matrix*, ed. D.W.L. Hukin, 161-186. Deerfield Beach, FL: Verlag Chemie.

Nikolic, V., and B. Zimmermann. 1968. Functional changes of the tarsal bones of ballet dancers. *Radovi Fakulteta u Zagrebu* 16: 131-146.

Pollack, G.H. 1990. *Muscles & molecules: Uncovering the principles of biological motion.* Seattle: Ebner & Sons.

Pratt, M. 1989. Strength, flexibility, and maturity in adolescent athletes. *American Journal of Diseases of Children* 143(5): 560-563.

Rosenbaum, D., and E.M. Hennig. 1995. The influence of stretching and warm-up exercises on Achilles tendon reflex activity. *Journal of Sports Sciences* 13(6): 481-490.

Sandstead, H.L. 1968. *The relationship of outward rotation of the humerus to baseball throwing velocity.* Unpublished master's thesis, Eastern Illinois University, Charleston, IL.

Sapega, A.A., T.C. Quedenfeld, R.A. Moyer, and R.A. Butler. 1981. Biophysical factors in range-of-motion exercise. *The Physician and Sportsmedicine* 9(12): 57-65.

Siff, M.C. 1993a. Exercise and the soft tissues. *Fitness and Sports Review International* 28(1): 32.

———. 1993b. Soft tissue biomechanics and flexibility. *Fitness and Sports Review International* 28(4): 127-128.

Simpson, D.G., W. Carver, T.K. Borg, and L. Terracio. 1994. Role of mechanical stimulation in the establishment and maintenance of muscle cell differentiation. *International Review of Cytology* 150: 69-94.

Snell, R.S. 1992. *Clinical anatomy for medical students*. Boston: Little, Brown.

Sutcliffe, M.C., and J.M. Davidson. 1990. Effect of static stretching on elastin production by porchine aortic smooth muscle cells. *Matrix* 10(3): 148-153.

Todd, T. 1985. The myth of the muscle-bound lifter. *NSCA Journal* 7(3): 37-41.

Wallis, E.L., and G.A. Logan. 1964. *Figure improvement and body conditioning through exercise*. Englewood Cliffs, NJ: Prentice-Hall.

Wang, K., R. McCarter, J. Wright, J. Beverly, and R. Ramirez-Mitchell. 1991. Regulation of skeletal muscle stiffness and elasticity by titin isoforms: A test of the segmental extension model of resting tension. *Proceedings of the National Academy of Science (USA)* 88(6): 7101-7105.

Williams, P.E., and G. Goldspink. 1971. Longitudinal growth of striated muscle fibres. *Journal of Cell Science* 9(3): 751-767.

Wilmore, J., and D.L. Costill. 1994. *Physiology of sport and exercise*. Champaign, IL: Human Kinetics.

Wilmore, J., R.B. Parr, R.N. Girandola, P. Ward, P.A. Vodak, T.V. Pipes, G.T. Romerom, and P. Leslie. 1978. Physiological alterations consequent to circuit weight training. *Medicine and Science in Sports* 10(2): 79-84.

Wolpaw, J.R., and J.S. Carp. 1990. Memory traces in spinal cord. *Trends in Neuroscience* 13(4): 137-142.

Zachazewski, J.E. 1990. Flexibility for sports. In *Sports physical therapy,* ed. B. Sanders, 201-238. Norwalk, CT: Appleton & Lange.

ABOUT THE AUTHOR

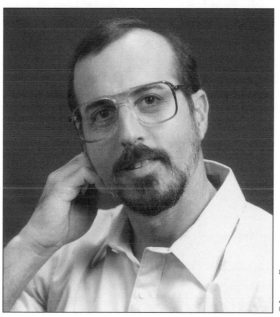

© Lenny Furman

A former gymnast, coach, and nationally certified men's gymnastics judge, Michael J. Alter is an expert on the subject of stretching. He is the author of *Science of Flexibility, Science of Stretching*, and the first edition of *Sport Stretch*.

Alter earned his MS in health education from Florida International University in 1976. He taught high school physical education and coached gymnastics for several years prior to his current position in Miami as a high school teacher.

Alter has been a guest lecturer at annual meetings across the country, including the 1994 Chiropractic Sports Science Symposium and the 1992 Scientific Meeting of the North American Society of Pediatric Exercise Medicine.

In his leisure time, Alter enjoys bicycling, listening to classical music, working out with weights, and studying sports medicine.

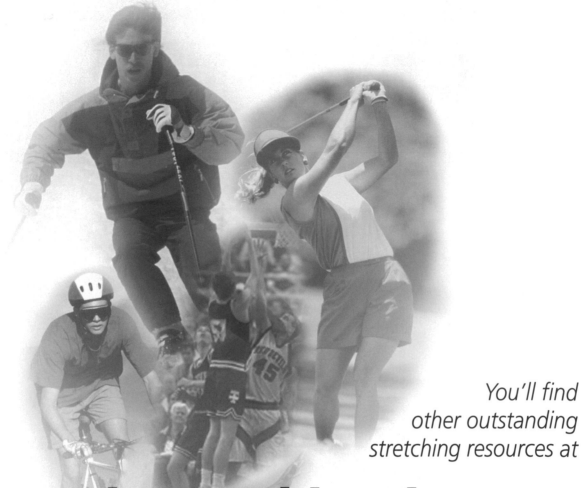